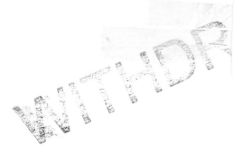

D1628166

ROYAL SOCIETY of MEDICINE Career Handbook

ST3 - Senior Doctor

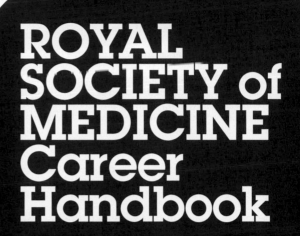

ROYAL SOCIETY of MEDICINE Career Handbook

ST3 - Senior Doctor

Kaji Sritharan MD(Res) MBBS FRCS

SpR in General Surgery, North West Thames Rotation,
London Deanery, Hon Research Fellow in Vascular Surgery
at Imperial College London

and **Muhunthan Thillai** BA MBBS MRCP PhD

Wellcome Trust Research Training Fellow and Honorary
Respiratory SpR at Imperial College London

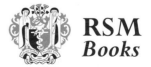

RSM *Books*

First published in Great Britain in 2012 by
Hodder Arnold, an imprint of Hodder Education, Hodder and Stoughton Ltd, a division of
Hachette UK
338 Euston Road, London NW1 3BH

http://www.hodderarnold.com

Hachette UK's policy is to use papers that are natural, renewable and recyclable products
and made from wood grown in sustainable forests. The logging and manufacturing
processes are expected to conform to the environmental regulations of the country of origin.

Whilst the advice and information in this book are believed to be true and accurate at
the date of going to press, neither the author[s] nor the publisher can accept any legal
responsibility or liability for any errors or omissions that may be made. In particular, (but
without limiting the generality of the preceding disclaimer) every effort has been made to
check drug dosages; however it is still possible that errors have been missed. Furthermore,
dosage schedules are constantly being revised and new side effects recognised. For these
reasons the reader is strongly urged to consult the drug companies' printed instructions, and
their websites, before administering any of the drugs recommended in this book.

British Library Cataloguing in Publication Data
A catalogue record for this book is available from the British Library

Library of Congress Cataloging-in-Publication Data
A catalog record for this book is available from the Library of Congress

ISBN-13 978-1-853-15929-9

1 2 3 4 5 6 7 8 9 10

Commissioning Editor: Caroline Makepeace
Project Editor: Joanna Silman
Production Controller: Joanna Walker
Cover Design: Helen Townson

Cover image © *Satum Stills/Science Photo Library*

The logo of the Royal Society of Medicine is a registered trade mark, which it has licensed to
Hodder Arnold.

Typeset in 10/14 Serifa Roman by Datapage India Pvt Ltd
Printed and bound by CPI Group (UK) Ltd., Croydon, CRO 4YY.

What do you think about this book? Or any other Hodder Arnold title?
Please visit our website: www.hodderarnold.com

To my Ammah and Appah – for giving me the courage and support to follow my dreams.

KS

Contents

Contributors

Alex Chan, Locum Consultant Paediatrician at Hillingdon Hospital (Chapter 13 Choosing your final job and the consultant interview)

Paul Gordon, Financial Advisor at MacArthur Gordon Ltd (Chapter 5 Managing your finances)

Andrew Papanikitas, GP trainee and PhD student (Chapter 4 General Practice)

Paul Thorpe, Consultant Spinal Surgeon at Taunton Hospital (Chapter 14 Now you're at the top...what next?

Acknowledgements

We are extremely grateful to Andrew Papanikitas, Paul Gordon, Alex Chan and Paul Thorpe for their authorship of chapters in this book. The chapters listed on p.8 were written entirely by them and this book would not have been possible without their hard work, adherence to guidelines and excellent personal insight into these areas.

We thank you all.

Introduction

Studying for an MBA at Harvard Business School is an opportunity only available to a select few. Only the very best, the most able and the hardest working make the cut. However, in the words of the school themselves, the MBA is not the final destination for these students, but *an important point of transition that prepares them for the opportunities that lie ahead.* Getting through your foundation years and the first years of specialist training is much like this. Only the very best will make it on to the specialist training programme of their choice but for those that do, this is just the beginning. The opportunities open to them will be immense and the choices and decisions that lie ahead often daunting.

Whether you want to be a successful full-time partner in a lucrative general practice, an inner city cardiologist or a part-time audiologist, getting to the top of your chosen specialty, especially in the current job market, can be a challenging process. The competition will be fierce as your colleagues all jostle for limited places in specialty training. Even once you have made it through this bottleneck, you will have to work hard to stand out from the crowd; above all you will have to decide how hard you are prepared to work and whether the sacrifices you need to make to get to where you want to go, are worth making.

The choices available to you are immense and the decisions you make will affect not only your career but also your life as a whole. Do you take time out of training to do research and should it be a three year lab-based PhD or a two year clinical MD? Do you accept that subspecialty training post in Edinburgh or are you better off applying for a Fellowship in New Zealand? Is it worth doing a teaching course or is your time better invested elsewhere?

Even choices that should be straightforward may, in reality, be difficult. How should you prepare for your ST3 interview? Should you continue as a salaried GP or try and look for a partnership? How do you manage your time both in and outside of work? Is it worth getting critical care cover or is life insurance enough?

In this second book, we have tried to address some of these more difficult decisions that you will be forced to make in your career as you become a more senior doctor. Not everyone wants to be a heart surgeon but whatever you choose, we hope that you will find the information in this book useful. Work hard, play hard and have a little faith in your own abilities. Everything else will fall into place.

Kaji Sritharan and Muhunthan Thillai
London

1

ST3 applications

Key aims of this chapter

- Choose the right specialty for you
- Define the application process
- Complete the application form.

Introduction

As a reader of this book you will probably have been a doctor for several years. Some of you will have decided that you are destined to be neurosurgeons, and will still be weighing up the merits of a career in anaesthetics versus one in respiratory medicine or general practice. For some, however, the right specialty will remain elusive. Importantly, every doctor is different and each will have different aspirations for the future. Moreover, these aspirations are likely to change over time as different priorities in your life become apparent.

Now is an important junction in your career and it is likely that the decisions you make at this point will significantly influence the course of your medical path. The aim of this chapter is to give you practical advice on how to choose a specialty and to guide you through the application process.

Which is the right specialty for me?

Making a career choice

No one can tell you which career is the right career for you, except you. There are, though, a number of factors that may influence your decision making and help you decide to pursue one specialty rather than another.

The current job market for your specialty

The competition for consultant posts at present for most hospital-based specialties is intense. Moreover, with the NHS struggling to manage debt (and therefore a general reluctance for Trusts to take on permanent staff), and a move towards centralisation of specialist services and to manage a greater proportion of patients in the community; the availability of consultant posts in hospital-based specialties is unlikely to improve dramatically in the future. That said, specialties may evolve and, as governments change, so may the plans for healthcare delivery. Therefore, although there may not be many posts in any one specialty now, in five or six years' time when you finish your training things may have opened up.

The competition for posts

If you feel that you have a 'weak' CV, you should take into account the competition for a specialty before applying, and you may even use the competition ratios to make a shortlist of the specialties that are appropriate for you (Table 1.1). Although the competition for a specialty will vary from

Table 1.1: Round 1 competition ratios for higher specialty training in 2011 (source: Modernising Medical Careers, www.mmc.nhs.uk)

Specialty	Posts available	Applications submitted	Competition ratio (applications per posts)
Acute medicine	109	351	3.22
Cardiology	94	607	6.46
Clinical pharmacology and therapeutics	15	21	1.40
Endocrinology and diabetes	85	265	3.12
Gastroenterology	94	441	4.69
General surgery	110	548	4.98
Geriatric medicine	115	307	2.67
Genitourinary medicine	42	74	1.76
Haematology	79	249	3.15
Neurology	43	161	3.74
Nuclear medicine	5	9	1.80
Palliative medicine	39	124	3.18
Plastic surgery	35	177	5.06
Psychiatry	219	550	2.51
Renal medicine	55	157	2.85
Respiratory medicine	120	408	3.40

year to year, certain specialties, such as general surgery, will always be popular and therefore competitive.

You should also compare your CV to the essential and desired qualities required within the 'person specification' for a post. Average candidates will meet *all* of the essential criteria and some of the desirable criteria, whereas excellent job candidates will meet *all* of the essential as well as *many* desirable qualities.

Opportunities to travel

If this is something that is important to you, certain specialties are more accommodating and easier to use as a base to travel from or with. For example, joining the military offers excellent surgical training opportunities and the ability to travel extensively, while becoming a GP will give you the flexibility to spend periods away doing voluntary work abroad.

Your research interests

During your undergraduate training, or indeed as a junior doctor, you may have had the opportunity to perform research. Some people flourish in this environment, while others are driven to despair. If you fall into the former category, you may want to take your research interests further and you should consider undertaking a PhD or MD at this stage or applying for an academic run-through position or lecturer post.

Your personality

Personality assessment tools, such as the Myers–Briggs test, are gaining in popularity in medicine, in particular in relation to developing management skills. In terms of determining your future career their role is less clear. Some research suggests that doctors within different specialties have different personality types, but all personality types are seen within all specialties. This suggests that, although determining your personality type may usefully facilitate discussion of the pros and cons of a career in relation to your personality, it by no means excludes you from any career, nor can it be used to find your perfect career. Another important fact is that both your personality type and your specialty are likely to change during the 40+ years of your career in medicine.

Deciding which specialty to apply to can be a difficult decision, one that you shouldn't try to make alone. Careers advice is available from your deanery, and your allocated educational or clinical supervisor and specialist royal college may also be able to help. In addition, you should speak to seniors within the specialty you are considering.

An approach to decision making

The UK Medical Careers website (www.medicalcareers.nhs.uk) advocates a four-stage approach to career planning.

Self-assessment

This is a process of understanding yourself – your strengths, interests (this is not necessarily the same as the things you are good at) and weaknesses – and it is helpful to write a list. Personality testing (e.g. a Myers–Briggs test) can also form a useful part of this process of self-discovery.

Additionally, list the factors that are important to you in terms of both your personal life (e.g. need for work–life balance, flexibility of hours, short training period) and work life (e.g. patient demographics, variety of caseload, clinical autonomy).

Career exploration

Review the list of specialties available or those that you have already shortlisted as a career and critically appraise each in terms of:

- what the job entails
- what it takes to succeed in that specialty (e.g. will you be spending weekends and evenings writing papers or book chapters?)
- the benefits or advantages
- the opportunities it presents (e.g. travel, research)
- the disadvantages.

Decision making

Having determined what drives you and evaluated the specialties available, you should be closer to arriving at a decision – or certainly have narrowed down your list of choices. Your ideal specialty should instil some excitement in you and provide you with a balance between your personal needs and your professional goals.

Plan implementation

Now that you have decided on a specialty (you may want to apply to more than one), you must plan how to reach your goal. This book intends to guide you through this journey. This chapter will give you advice about the application process, Chapter 2 discusses how you can achieve success at interview, and Chapter 12 gives guidance on how to make the most of your specialty training – including developing your CV and portfolio. The latter should demonstrate your commitment to, and enthusiasm for, the specialty you have chosen.

How do I apply?

Where to apply

Applications to specialty training programmes are managed by either a single 'lead deanery' or one of the royal colleges on behalf of the deaneries. The process of application is coordinated on a national level. Thus only one application is required for any one specialty, and on your application form you will be asked to rank in order your preferred regions for training. The exceptions to this are the smaller specialties, where they may not be a delegated 'lead deanery' or appointed college. In this situation, application for a training programme is made directly to the deanery advertising the post.

For all specialties the process of application is online and you can apply to as many specialties as you wish provided you meet the eligibility and competency level criteria for the post.

The person specification

This outlines the essential and desirable criteria required in order to apply for a training programme. The specifications are readily available for all specialties through the Medical Specialty Training (England) website (www.mmc.nhs.uk) from November of any given application year.

You should study the person specification for your specialty early in your medical career, ideally well before the specialty application process (i.e. as a foundation or core trainee). It should serve as a benchmark and focus for the development of your CV and portfolio. Thinking about this early will stand you in good stead for applying to specialty positions, as your CV and portfolio are likely to have a clearer direction.

Types of post

There are two main types of specialty training programme:

● 'Run-through' training is where there is seamless progression from core training (referred to as ST1/ST2) to specialty training (ST3 to ST5/6 typically) on the proviso that the necessary competency requirements are met.

- 'Uncoupled' training programmes are where, following two years of core training (CT1/CT2) (three years in some specialties), there is open competition into specialty training (ST3 to ST5/6 typically) posts.

Academic clinical fellowships (ACFs) offer run-through training in specialties that are normally uncoupled; see www.nihrtcc.nhs.uk/intetacatrain for more details.

The endpoint of a specialty training programme is the certificate of completion of training (CCT) or equivalent, which will grant you entry on to the General Medical Council's specialist or GP register. For those who have undertaken a non-standard training, the endpoint is the certificate of eligibility for specialist or general practice registration (CESR) (Box 1.1).

What are FTSTAs?

Fixed-term specialty training appointments (FTSTAs) are one-year stand-alone training posts that exist in run-through specialties such as neurosurgery and paediatrics. They are useful to undertake if you want to experience a particular specialty before committing to it, or if you need more time to fulfill the entry requirements for ST training or make your CV more competitive before applying. It is well worth remembering that, if you are successful in obtaining an FTSTA position, your chances of subsequently obtaining a run-through post at ST2 will be low, as there will be very few of these posts available.

When should I apply?

The *first round* of recruitment into specialty training in the UK kicks off in late November for CT1/2 posts and CT3 posts in psychiatry and

It is possible to train flexibly (i.e. part-time) if you can demonstrate that training on a full-time basis is not feasible or practicable for you, for clear reasons such as a disability, illness or carer responsibilities. The same competency requirements as for full-time trainees exist in order to attain your certificate of completion of training (CCT) or certificate of eligibility for specialist registration (CESR), but the length of training to achieve these competencies will be longer.

Box 1.1 Flexible training

emergency medicine and ST1/4 run-through posts – with a deadline for closure of applications in mid-December and interviews and offers made by early March. Applications for all uncoupled ST3 posts, previously unadvertised CT2 posts and CT2 posts in anaesthestics start in early February, with interviews held in April and offers made shortly thereafter.

The exact timing of the application process may vary subtly among the different recruiting offices, but all will in general follow the national timetable. Each recruitment office should publicise the timeline of the recruitment process on their website well in advance, so this will allow you to plan submitting your application, and ear-marking time off for potential interviews. Posts will typically be advertised for a minimum of four weeks on the recruiting office and NHS Jobs websites.

Each recruitment office oversees:

- publicising the timeline for their recruitment process
- advertising posts
- giving guidance on completing application forms
- receiving and shortlisting online applications
- coordinating the interview process
- advising you about the outcome of your application.

The recruitment process for academic clinical fellowships is run by the National Institute for Health Research Trainees Coordinating Centre (www.nihrtcc.nhs.uk). It usually starts in mid-October, with the deadline for applications in mid-November, and interviews conducted and offers given by the end of January. Similarly, the recruitment process into general practice also differs from that for other specialties. The application process for GPs opens in mid-November and closes in early December. Applicants shortlisted for GP training are then required to undertake a marked test and attend a GP assessment centre, with offers issued by early March.

Who can apply?

In order to apply for a specialty training programme or post you must meet the eligibility criteria by either the start of the post or by closure of the application date. These criteria include the following:

- You must meet the national person specifications for the post.
- You must be registered with the General Medical Council (GMC) or the General Dental Council (GDC).

- You must be entitled to work in the United Kingdom. UK and EEA nationals are eligible to apply to specialty training posts. Non-UK or non-EEA nationals with limited leave to remain in the UK, whose employment requires a Tier 2 visa, are subject to the resident labour market test and will be considered only if there are no suitable UK or EEA national candidates for the post; so they may apply in round 2 (see below) but not round 1 of the application process.
- There must be evidence of your English language skills. If your undergraduate training was not in English, you will need to provide evidence of English language skills, such as your International English Language Testing System (IELTS) score. If your undergraduate training was in English, but not in the UK, you will need written evidence to verify this.
- For ST3 entry to the medical specialties you will need to have passed Part 2 written examination but not the PACES (Part 2 clinical examination) component of the MRCP(UK) exam at the time of receiving an offer for a post. You should have completed all components of the exam before taking up the position. For ST3 entry to the surgical specialties, you should have successfully completed all components of the MRCS (see Chapter 3).
- To be eligible to apply for ST1 and CT1 posts you cannot have held a post in the specialty you are applying to for more than 18 months (exceptions being chemical pathology, histopathology, medical microbiology, virology, and public health). There is no limit on experience for eligibility for entry at ST2/CT2/ST3/ST4.
- You must show evidence of achievement of foundation competences. This can be demonstrated in three ways:
  - confirmation of the name of your foundation school if you are currently in foundation training
  - award of a foundation achievement of competence document (FACD)
  - submission of alternative evidence of completion of acquisition of foundation competencies.

Advice about applications can be obtained (usually by email) from individual deaneries or from the Department of Health's Medical Education and Training Programme (England) national support helpdesk (see the end of this chapter). All emails should be answered within 48 hours or, if further information or investigation is required, within five working days.

Round 2 of recruitment

Round 2 of the application process mops up jobs not filled in round 1 and includes new posts that have arisen during the year. It starts when round 1 has finished (typically in early February for CT1/ST1 posts, and at the end of March for ST3 posts) and can extend until the end of October. This presents another opportunity to apply, should you have failed to secure a place in round 1.

You can also apply to posts in round 2 if you have already accepted a post in round 1, however you will need to make the deanery you are applying to aware that you have accepted a post in round 1, as well as the deanery you have accepted the post from that you are applying elsewhere. The former will not prejudice your application. If you are successful you will need to work any notice period before taking up the new post. Unlike in round 1, non-UK/EEA nationals can apply for posts in this round, but priority will still be given to UK/EEA applicants.

Longlisting and shortlisting

For most specialties, shortlisting is based on the content of the application form in relation to the nationally advertised person specification for a post. It may be preceded by a process of longlisting, whereby all candidates who meet the essential criteria of the person specification are put to one side and then shortlisted (i.e. scored and ranked), with the top-scoring individuals being invited to interview. Typically, more people are invited to interview than there are posts available.

In certain specialties, namely general practice and public health, in addition to the application form, recruitment is based on performance at an assessment centre. In other specialties, all candidates may be invited to interview.

Interviews

This topic is covered in detail in Chapter 2. Importantly, once an offer of interview is made, you will be given a limited time (typically just 48 hours) to confirm whether you will be attending the interview or assessment centre.

Job offers

From 2012, there is to be UK-wide coordination between the UK health departments, royal colleges and deaneries for all first offers in round 1, with offers for CT1/ST1 posts issued by the beginning of March and by mid–late May for CT2/ST3 positions. Applicants will thus be able to accept, reject or hold a round 1 offer until after all round 1 first offers have been made.

You can only hold one offer at any one time, but it is possible to 'upgrade' an offer. This means that, if you hold or accept an offer that is a lower preference (from your original choices) than your first choice, you will have the option to either hold the post you have been allocated or accept the offer with upgrades. If you choose to accept with upgrades, you may still receive a better offer (a higher preference) from the same specialty if one becomes available.

As previously, the timeframe to respond to an offer is 48 hours. This period includes weekends and bank holidays, so it is imperative that you check your emails on a daily basis as a lack of response to an offer will be viewed as a rejection. It is vital that you also check your junk mail folder in case the emails are sent there.

Offers are made on the premise that you have not accepted any other offer and that you have withdrawn from the application process. The exceptions to this rule are:

- Academic Clinical Fellowships ACFs – you can still apply to an ACF if you have accepted a run-through training programme
- CT2 or CT3 posts in emergency medicine and psychiatry
- a fixed-term specialty training appointment (FTSTA) – you can apply to continue to run-through training posts or for uncoupled training programmes, but you cannot apply to other FTSTAs or one year of training posts.

Also, from 2012, certain nationally coordinated specialties – including anaesthetics (West Midlands Deanery), neurosurgery (Yorkshire & Humber Deanery) and public health (East Midlands Deanery) – will use the UK offers system (UKOFFS) to make offers. So, if you are applying to any of these specialties managed by these deaneries you will need to be registered online with UKOFFS in order to receive news of your application; this needs to be done within two weeks of receiving an email from them. For all other specialties, it will be the lead deanery or royal college that will issue any offers. *From 2013, UKOFFS will be the only portal for receiving job offers across all specialties.* Importantly, through UKOFFS once you have accepted an offer no further offers will be made to you.

What if I don't get an offer?

You should request feedback from your recruiting office, if it has not already be given online. Ask for your shortlisting score – including your rank, total score, number of applicants, and score required to be eligible for interview. Feedback regarding your application can also be requested.

In addition, if you attended an interview, your interview score, overall rank, number of interviewees and rank required to obtain an offer should be requested. You can also ask for copies of your interview score sheets. In accordance with the Data Protection Act, this information should be provided within 40 days.

What if you do not get a training post?

Even after round 1 and 2 of specialty recruitment, deaneries may continue to advertise any unfilled posts until late October. If you do not get a post into specialty training, you have a number of options:

- Apply for a post as locum appointed for training (LAT) or locum appointed for service (LAS), or a Trust grade (non-training grade) post. A LAT can be counted towards the time required for CCT.
- Consider a period in research (see Chapter 7).
- Consider a position abroad (see Chapter 11).

You can seek advice about your career development from a number of sources: your educational supervisor, clinical tutor or director of medical education at your hospital; the royal colleges' specialty organisations or trainee groups; and the British Medical Association's careers guidance service.

The application form

What does the form require?

The application form is in electronic format and should be completed and submitted online. You will need to register with the application portal, which can take up to 30 minutes. *Note that late applications will not be accepted*, so you should note when the application process opens for your specialty and aim to apply early to avoid last-minute glitches with the system as everyone try to get their applications in at the last minute.

Application forms are geared towards assessing whether you meet the national person specification for the post. Look at this in relation to your specialty, so you can tailor and focus your application accordingly.

The application form has two parts (a sample can be found at www. mmc.nhs.uk). The first part is generic (the same for all posts) and asks for personal information. The second part is specific to a specialty. The online application form takes on average an hour to complete, but it can take several days or weeks for you to formulate answers to the questions, get feedback and tweak your answers to get them to the point where you are happy with them. All shortlisters and interviewers will have access to your application form in its entirety with the exception of the equal opportunities and personal information section.

Completing your application

- Plan ahead! Establish early when the application process for your specialty opens and closes.
- Contact your referees early and make sure they are agreeable to supporting your application and can provide a reference within the given time frame. You need three referees who have supervised you clinically within the past three years (they can be different if you are applying to more than one specialty/post); or, if you have had a career break, your two most recent clinical supervisors.
- Think about the person specification for your specialty and gather examples (e.g. audits, research, presentations) and evidence (e.g. course and meeting attendance and exam certificates, publications) that you can use in your application and which demonstrate you meet the person specification.
- There will be questions on the skills you possess (e.g. team-player, organised, good communicator, leader). You should try to give examples to illustrate your point within each question (Box 1.2).

The STAR technique is a useful strategy to use to answer competency-based questions. It is based on structuring your answer into three parts: the Situation/Task, Action and Result.

- **Situation/Task** describes a scenario and gives context for the action. This should be concise and relevant to the question being answered (any clinical information should be kept to the essentials). Do not use more than 25 per cent of the allocated word count on this part, as it carries few marks.
- **Action** should form the bulk (75 per cent) of the answer and should demonstrate and emphasise the skill or personal attribute being tested. Your answer should be personal; i.e. it should be about what you did and, importantly, why.
- **Result** is a brief (25 per cent of the word count) explanation of the outcome of your actions and what you accomplished or learnt.

Box 1.2 Tips on answering questions

- Review your work-based assessments, CV and extracurricula activities and come up with examples (ideally original ones) that could be used to answer these questions.
- Think of examples to questions that are unique, personal and interesting.
- Answers and examples should demonstrate your enthusiasm and commitment to the specialty you are applying to.
- Try to end your answers to questions on a positive note. There is no point in describing a clinical situation where you demonstrate great communication skills but the patient dies.

- Draft your answers within a separate document. This makes corrections easier and you can simply paste your answers into the online application form when the time comes.
- Check the word count allowed and stick to it. If any of your answers are over the limit the question at best will be ignored and at worst the application will be automatically rejected.
- Get opinions on your proposed answers from medical and non-medical friends and colleagues. Ask them for honest, constructive feedback.
- Before submitting your application, ensure you both spell- and grammar-check your answers.

Sources of further information

Academic clinical fellowships: www.nihrtcc.nhs.uk/intetacatrain

Medical Education and Training Programme (England) support helpdesk: medicalspecialtysupport@dh.gsi.gov.uk

Modernising Medical Careers: www.mmc.nhs.uk

National Institute of Health Research Trainees Coordinating Centre: www.nihrtcc.nhs.uk

Quick Guide to Recruitment in 2012: published October 2011 by the Department of Health's Medical Education and Training Programme team

Reference Guide for Postgraduate Specialty Training in the UK (Gold Guide, 4th edn): published June 2010 by the four UK Health Departments

UK Medical Careers: www.medicalcareers.nhs.uk

2

ST3 interviews

Key aims of this chapter

- Give an overview of the interview process
- Give advice on how to prepare for the interview and perform well on the day
- Give an overview of interview styles and formats.

Introduction

The interview is the final hurdle and, although you may be ecstatic that you've been shortlisted, the game is far from over. The interview requires an immense amount of preparation and should be approached like an exam. Moreover, the most common reason for people to come unstuck on the day is a lack of preparation or a lack of the right preparation. This chapter aims to guide you through the interview process, give you advice on how to prepare, and tips on how to perform well on the day. Much of this information is applicable to interviews at all stages in your medical career, but some information – particularly regarding the types of interview format – are specifically designed for ST3 and above.

Interview basics

Organising your interview

Most interviews are organised at deanery level, with a smaller variable number run by NHS Trusts. Typically more people are invited to interview than there are posts and this is to ensure that all the jobs are filled. Once shortlisted, you will be notified of the date, time and location of the interview – either by email (so keep an eye on your junk email folder) or by post. Details of the interviewing process and scoring scheme should be available to you at your request, and you should aim to get the lowdown on the format well ahead of the interview day. This will guide your preparation.

You are usually given at least five days' notice of the interview. However, it can be far less, for example if someone drops out and a gap arises. So if you are relatively confident that you have a good chance of being short-listed, it is worthwhile noting the dates of the interviews for that specialty (found on the deanery website) and gently starting to prepare. You should also inform your current employer or colleagues of your potential interview dates, so they are not left short on the day and can make the necessary plans to cover your absence.

As before, you have a limited timeframe in which to confirm your intention to attend the interview. Check with the deanery that you have confirmed your attendance if you don't get an email acknowledging your response.

If you are fortunate to be in the position where you have been interviewed and have accepted a job in a different post, you should out of courtesy let the deanery know. You will be withdrawn from the interview list, which will give someone else the chance to be interviewed. You should also inform the deanery if you have a clash of interview dates – for example, if are invited to interview in two different specialties. When this occurs it may be possible to move interview times/dates, but you need to give the deanery as much notice as possible.

If you don't receive a response to your application, this suggests that you haven't been shortlisted – only successful candidates are contacted. However, it is worth contacting your centre of application (lead deanery or royal college) if you think that perhaps the invitation for interview may have been 'lost'. Moreover, if you think you have been unfairly not shortlisted, there are complaints/appeals procedures in place and you have the right to ask for feedback (in particular your shortlisting score).

Preparation before the interview

Some deaneries (e.g. Yorkshire) offer mock interviews, so it is worth contacting the deanery you have been shortlisted for to see whether this service exists. Mock interviews are usually held either at the deanery itself or within education centres affiliated to the deanery. The earlier you ask about these opportunities the better, as places fill up rapidly.

The interview is about demonstrating to the panel that not only do you meet the person specification for the post, but that you are the best person for the job. Your responses to questions should be structured, and this means you should think about potential questions and answers before the interview. Ask your colleagues, your educational supervisor and your consultant trainer for interview advice and, more importantly, interview practice. Ask for feedback about your performance as this is the ideal opportunity to correct any annoying mannerisms or poor technique.

In addition, review the essential criteria and person specification for the post, your CV, your strengths and weaknesses and your portfolio – as these will be the focus of the interview. You can predict more than 80 per cent of the questions that arise in the interview, so write a list of these and think about your approach to the answers.

What should I take to the interview?

You will be told by your deanery what you need to take. The deanery is required to verify your identity, registration, qualifications and status with respect to working, and the following are usually required (this is not an exhaustive list):

- proof of identity, such as a valid passport or official photo ID (original plus two copies)
- two recent, passport-size photographs with your name written clearly on the back of each
- your original GMC certificate for the current year + photocopies
- your original degree certificate and relevant postgraduate qualifications, including evidence of all qualifications listed on your application form (with official translations if the original is not in English) + photocopies
- evidence of educationally approved posts held as stated in your application form
- evidence of skills in written and spoken English
- verified evidence of competences cited on your application form (i.e. your portfolio)
- evidence of eligibility to take up employment in the UK, including evidence of immigration status if a non-UK/EEA applicant, or appropriate passport, birth certificate or naturalisation papers for UK/EEA applicants + photocopies

- evidence of achievement of foundation and core competencies (i.e. your portfolio).

If for any reason you cannot provide the above/required documents you should obtain a certified copy and contact the deanery prior to your interview. Failure to produce any of the requested documents may result in you not being interviewed.

Can I claim expenses?

Essential costs of attending the interview can be claimed (Box 2.1).

It should be possible to claim travelling expenses for attending the interview. Expense forms are usually available at interview. Some deaneries ask for confirmation that you will be claiming for travel expenses in advance of the interview date, or require a request in writing, especially if overnight accommodation is required. Costs are paid in accordance with the Whitley Council terms and conditions, and receipts for costs incurred need to be produced.

Box 2.1 Claiming travel expenses

General interview tips for the day

First impressions in any interview count. Some general advice is given below to help steer you away from trouble.

- The dress code for interviews is 'smart and conservative'. Men should wear a suit and tie; women similarly should wear a suit/jacket. Now is not the time to stand out from the crowd!
- Arrive early – at least 30–45 minutes beforehand.
  - If you are running late you should telephone through as it may be possible to reorganise the timing. If you just turn up late, you may not be interviewed at all.
  - If you are driving, make sure there will be parking facilities, and that you have enough change for a meter.
  - If taking public transport, leave plenty of time for unexpected cancellations or delays.
- Try not to make plans for after the interview. Interview schedules often run behind time, so if you need to be somewhere shortly after the interview, you are likely to be late.

The interview structure

This will vary across deaneries, specialties and your level of entry. Most postgraduate medical interviews are structured or semi-structured, which means that all candidates will be asked the same questions or questions with a similar theme. So it really is in your best interest not to divulge questions to candidates awaiting interview on the same day. It is also worth bearing in mind that, although the opening question may be the same for all candidates, depending on your response, further probing or follow-up questions are premitted and will vary between candidates.

Interviews tend to take an objective structured clinical exam (OSCE) format. The number of stations will vary between deaneries and specialties, ranging between two and six. Within each station there will usually be two or three panel members. Generally, at ST entry, interviews will last for a minimum of 30 minutes, and each station will last a minimum of 10 minutes. You should expect to cover three to four questions within each station; and importantly, the stations can vary considerably in format, from structured questions and a written assessment to a presentation or critique of a paper. You should determine the nature of the interview beforehand, as this will be essential to guide your preparation.

Before the interview, all members of the panel will have had access to your anonymised application form, excluding any equal opportunities or personal data. The interview panel members will have met with the lay-chairman 30–45 minutes before the interviews start, to allocate stations and discuss which of the preset questions each of them is going to ask. Often one examiner will ask questions for the first half and then they will swap over roles.

Your interview experience

- The panel members will introduce themselves and might offer you a handshake.
- Remember, most interviewers will form an opinion of you in the first 90 seconds, so make a good impression from the beginning. No one else will believe in you if you don't believe in yourself. Be positive and confident (but not over-confident) – you have been invited to the interview, so you have a clear chance of securing the job.
- Listen carefully to the question asked and ensure that you understand it. If you don't understand the question, ask the interviewer to repeat it. Be careful, however, to do this only once or twice during the interview as it can annoy some interviewers.

- Don't rush into answering question. When you hear a question, even if it is something you can easily answer and are fully prepared, take a second or two before you start. It is often the first sentence that leads the discussion relating to that part of the interview, and it is surprising how many people, even though they know the subject matter very well, start badly and are never able to recover.
- Answer the question asked! Do not go off on a tangent, or answer a different question you would have liked to be asked.
- Be honest in your responses. The panel are looking to employ a future colleague, so clear enthusiasm, commitment and honesty are essential.
- Direct each response to the person who asked the question, but make sure you don't ignore the rest of the panel.
- Avoid sounding as though you have rote-learnt answers to questions. Even if you have a well-rehearsed response to a question, pause and deliver your reply as naturally as possible.
  - Structure your answers. Don't ramble on, but focus on the key points the interviewer is looking for and give them in order of importance. The interviewer is looking for a clear thought process, so don't take three minutes to say something that can be said in one minute. This will limit the number of questions you get asked.
  - If you are asked to give an opinion, it is useful to initially give both sides of the argument. However, don't sit on the fence. You will undoubtedly be challenged and you should be able to defend your stance, while demonstrating an ability to listen to other perspectives.
  - Where possible/appropriate, you should try to demonstrate reflective practice. For example, when asked to describe a situation, structure your response by giving some information regarding the setting, describe your involvement and the skills you called upon, and reflect on the outcome in terms of what you have learnt from the experience and how you might tackle the same or similar situation in the future.
- Throughout the interview maintain good eye-contact with all members of the panel.
- Avoid fidgeting. Place your hands firmly on your knees throughout the interview if this helps.
- During the interview you may hear bells or knocks on the door indicating the times. Do not be put off by these. Keep talking until someone tells you that the interview has finished.
- If a question or station seems to go badly, try to put it behind you and remain calm – the odds are that you haven't done as badly as you feel

you have. You will be asked many questions, and doing badly – or at least thinking you've done badly – in a few may not impact significantly on your overall performance.

● At the termination of a station you will be asked by the coordinator to wait and then will be directed to the next station.

● Expect to be tested to your limit and put under pressure. This is one way in which examiners try to distinguish one good candidate from another.

● At the end of the interview you may be asked whether you have any questions. You will not be penalised for not having any questions (politely say no – the safest option). If you ask a question, beware that the information has not been given previously or elsewhere (e.g. in the person specification), or that it demonstrates ignorance.

● Once you have finished all the stations you will be allowed to leave the interview room. Remember to thank the interviewer(s).

How will I be marked?

At each station, each panel member will mark the sections discussed in that station separately from his/her co-panel members according to the person specification for the post, and have the opportunity to add comments to justify the score given. There will therefore be at least two sets of marks for each station.

After the interviews have been completed, all the marks for each of the candidates are collated and the aggregate score given by all panel members is used to give a final score. Using this score, candidates will be ranked. It is not possible for the marks to be changed as they are collected from the panel members by the administrative coordinator at regular intervals during the interviews and are collated into the accumulated scores.

In the briefing discussion before the interviews begin, the panel members may decide that certain questions are so important that, should the candidate not answer them correctly, he or she will be 'red-carded'. This often relates to clinical scenarios where the panel feel that the candidate's clinical experience, if a question is not answered appropriately, would deem him or her unsuitable for the post. The panel members and the lay-chairman between them establish clear guidelines as to the grounds on which a red card can be issued. Thus after the interview when the marks are looked at, although a candidate may have been ranked high enough to be offered a job, if he or she has been red-carded in any section of the interview, they will be automatically eliminated from the selection.

The role of references

References can be unstructured (free text) or structured. In the latter, your referee may be asked a number of questions including those regarding your clinical ability, future potential, team-working skills and interaction with patients and colleagues – attributes as outlined by the GMC's document *Good Medical Practice*. The references are not seen by the panel members and are viewed only by the lay-chairman. A key role of the lay-chairman is to review the written references, to ensure there is nothing therein to deem the candidate unappointable. The references will also be reviewed by the employer if you are successful at interview.

Interview questions

As mentioned earlier, interviews tend to take on an Objective Structure Clinical Examination OSCE format, as this has been shown to be a fair, reproducible and transparent method to select the most appropriate candidate. Moreover, the structured marking system allows for little variability between examiners. OSCE stations aim to assess a specific set of criteria that you will be given the opportunity to demonstrate through the way you answer a given question or respond to a given task.

The interview panel will be looking to ensure that you meet the essential criteria as well as possess specific qualities as stated in the person specification for the post (Box 2.2). This will be achieved through assessment over a number of stations, each of which will take a slightly different slant. As part of your interview preparation you should consider questions that are commonly asked and prepare answers to each according to your own experiences.

- Clinical knowledge and expertise:
  - appropriate knowledge base
  - capacity to apply sound clinical judgement to problems
  - ability to prioritise clinical need
  - awareness of the basics of managing acutely ill patients.

- Vigilance and situational awareness:
  - capacity to be alert to dangers or problems
  - capacity to monitor developing situations and anticipate issues.

(Continued)

(Continued)

- Coping with pressure:
  - capacity to operate under pressure
  - initiative and resilience to cope with setbacks and adapt to rapidly changing circumstances
  - awareness of own limitations and when to ask for help.

- Managing Others and Team Involvement
  - capacity to work cooperatively with others
  - ability to work effectively in multi-professional teams
  - leadership skills.

- Problem solving and decision making:
  - capacity to solve problems
  - ability to make decisions.

- Empathy and sensitivity:
  - capacity to take in others' perspectives and treat others with understanding
  - sees patients as people.

- Communication skills:
  - demonstrates clarity in written/spoken communication
  - adapts language as appropriate to the situation
  - able to build rapport, listen, persuade and negotiate.

- Organisation and planning:
  - capacity to organise oneself, prioritise own work and organise ward rounds
  - demonstrates punctuality, preparation and self-discipline
  - possesses basic IT skills.

- Professional integrity and respect for others:
  - capacity to take responsibility for own actions
  - demonstrates a non-judgemental approach towards others
  - displays honesty, integrity, awareness of confidentiality and ethical issues
  - possesses delegation skills.

- Learning and personal development:
  - demonstrates interest and realistic insight in the specialty
  - demonstrates self-awareness.

Box 2.2 Qualities the panel will be looking for

There can be a great variation in the types of station encountered, but they usually include two or more of the following:

- portfolio-based interviews
- research, teaching and publications
- clinical governance, audit and management
- clinical experience
- behavioural questions, addressing aspects of the person specification such as team-working, ethics etc.
- communication skills
- presentations
- practical skills
- critical analysis
- group discussion.

Portfolio-based interviews

Portfolio-based stations are commonplace and can be used to assess a number of aspects of your person specification including your career progression and learning and development. You will be expected to bring your portfolio to the interview (remember it should not contain any patient identifiable data). Within these stations you may simply be asked to hand over your portfolio for review by the examiner, or you may be asked questions centred on your portfolio. The aim of questioning in this context is to substantiate the evidence contained within your portfolio. You should know your portfolio inside out and be prepared to answer questions on all parts of it, including statements made in relation to your portfolio in your application form (Box 2.3).

A common opening question is: 'Talk me through your portfolio.' This is a gift of a question. However, it is also a very easy question to answer badly. Remember that you only have a limited amount of time, so structure your answer – demonstrating focus in your career pathway to date, commitment to your specialty, and drive. You should summarise your clinical experience and highlight your strengths and achievements and outline where you see yourself in the near future.

Other frequently asked questions include: 'What have you learnt whilst putting together your portfolio?', 'Why do you think it's important to maintain a portfolio?', and 'What are your strengths and weaknesses as evidenced by your portfolio?'

Your portfolio should be your own work. It should be logically presented and include the following:

- A list of competences required to successfully complete the foundation programme.
- Records of meetings with your educational supervisor.
- A personal development plan (PDP) including career planning.
- Presented evidence:
  - exam certificates
  - certificates of course/lecture/tutorial attendance
  - posters presented at learned meetings
  - presentations, including at Journal Clubs
  - abstracts and papers (full texts)
  - audit projects (full texts)
  - a reflective log of activities and experience
  - a Logbook of clinical activity or record of achieved competencies signed by your trainer (e.g. procedures or operations).
- Work-based assessments (WBAs):
  - 360-degree assessments or mini-PATS
  - DOPS
  - a mini-CEX
  - case-based discussions
  - procedure-based assessments.

CEX, clinical evaluation exercise; DOPS, direct observation of procedural skills; PATS, peer assessment tools.

Box 2.3 The contents of your portfolio

You may be asked questions aimed at establishing your commitment to the specialty, or the deanery you have applied to. Examples are: 'Why have you applied to this deanery?', 'How have you demonstrated your commitment and aptitude for this specialty?', and 'Why this specialty?' The latter may be evidenced by previous posts held, 'tasters', membership of the relevant learned societies, attendance at courses or meetings relevant to your specialty, and specialty-specific research/audit. You should bring these to the fore in the interview.

Research, publications and teaching

You could encounter an individual 'research, teaching and publications' station, but questions on these topics may also be covered elsewhere in the interview, such as your portfolio station. The obvious exception to this is an application for a post in academic medicine.

Research

Discussion in this part will centre on any academic research you have previously conducted or are currently performing. You may have completed an intercalated BSc or a BSc before entering medical school. Others may have done an MSc, performed research as part of their elective, or completed an MD/PhD.

A common opening question is: 'Tell us about your research experience.' As with any question, you should pause and give a structured response rather than rush into an answer. Here, a chronological and clear description of your experience to date is expected and you should be prepared to answer questions on your research. For example, if you mention laboratory-based research you may be asked about laboratory methods. In addition, you should be prepared to answer research-related questions, such as: 'How has this research impacted on clinical practice?', 'Tell me about a paper which changed your management of a patient', or 'What have you gained from your research?'

Publications

Presentations and publications will, in the main, be derived from research or audit you have conducted, individual case reports or clinical reviews. When completing the application form you should read the section on publications very carefully. Although it may fill the space on the form, to list publications including abstracts and letters or papers that are as yet unpublished can irritate some interviewers. At interview, interviewers will want to know about those that have actually been accepted or published.

Common questions in this area are: 'Out of all your publications, which one is the most important?', and 'Which one have you made the greatest contribution to?' When answering this question, you should acknowledge to the panel the level of your contribution. Even if you have not performed all the work yourself, you should have a clear understanding of all parts of the paper (e.g. methods of cell culture, RNA extraction). Other associated questions that may arise include those on evidenced-based medicine, such as: 'What is evidence-based medicine?' or 'Do you practice evidence-based medicine?'; and those on research methodology, for example: 'What are the different levels of evidence?', 'What do you understand by the term randomised controlled trial (RCT)?', or 'Tell me about a case where EBM influenced the management of your patient'.

Teaching

By this point in your career you should have some teaching experience. At interview common opening questions are: 'Tell us what experience you have of teaching', or 'What are the characteristics of a good trainer?'

Most people will have had experience of teaching undergraduates, and this may be lecturing on revision courses and preparing medical students for their exams or during their attachment to your firm. A few interviewees may also have experience of teaching postgraduates – colleagues, and other healthcare professionals (e.g. nurses, physiotherapists, ambulance crews). Your teaching experience may also extend to developing or organising postgraduate and undergraduate courses, and it is essential that you make sure you discuss these in detail during the interview. It is also useful when answering this question to give some idea of your time commitment to teaching. For example, you may teach medical students for two hours each week.

Questions following from this may require discussion of your own teaching strengths or weaknesses, your preferred teaching methods, and the attributes of a good teacher. Importantly, teaching experience is not just about delivering teaching but also about developing teaching skills. You may have attended a course such as 'Teaching the teachers', or have undertaken a medical education degree. Bring this into the discussion.

Clinical governance, audit and management

Clinical governance

In this station, clinical governance is often dealt with using case scenarios, and the example used will be different for different specialties. An example in surgery may be: 'What would you do if a swab has been left in the wound and the swab count is incorrect at the end of the procedure?' In general medicine, similar scenarios may relate to your management of patients who have been given the wrong medication – either the wrong drug or the wrong dose – or a drug interaction. Examples are: 'A patient who has a penicillin allergy is accidentally administered penicillin. How would tackle this?', or 'How do you explain to a patient that a postoperative complication has arisen?'

Note that the General Medical Council gives clear guidance within *Good Medical Practice* regarding the management of adverse events at work:

> *If a patient under your care has suffered harm or distress, you must act immediately to put matters right, if that is possible. You should offer an apology and explain fully and promptly to the patient what has happened, and the likely short-term and long-term effects. ... Patients who complain about the care or treatment they have received have a right to expect a prompt, open, constructive and honest response including an explanation and, if appropriate, an apology. You must not allow a patient's complaint to affect adversely the care or treatment you provide or arrange.*

All of these types of clinical scenario also require you to mention critical incident reporting. You should be prepared to answer related questions such as: 'What happens to the critical incident form after you have completed it?', 'What feedback is given as a result of a clinical incident?', and 'Give an example where the outcome of action you took in response to a clinical mistake/error made you reassess how you would deal with similar events in the future.'

You should have a reasonable knowledge of how clinical governance works and importantly demonstrate how you have participated in it in your career to date. So be prepared to give examples (e.g. in relation to risk management, audit, and keeping up to date).

Audit

You should have either initiated or been involved in an audit by this stage in your career. Audit questions will usually start along the lines of: 'Discuss one of the audits you have done', 'Tell me about your most interesting audit', or 'Tell me about your most valuable audit'.

You will be expected to discuss one audit you have undertaken, why you undertook it, what results you obtained and, of course, what has been done to close the loop and the impact of the audit on your clinical practice. Further questions may include: 'What is clinical audit?', 'What are the benefits of audit?', and 'How does audit differ from research?'

Management

Management for junior trainees is a difficult topic to discuss at interview since most trainees will have had little experience of management at this stage. In this part of the interview, discussions on management are far more likely to focus on specific areas such as the National Institute for Health and

Clinical Excellence (NICE), the European Working Time Directive (EWTD), Modernising Medical Careers (MMC) etc. Examples are: 'What is NICE?', 'Describe one NICE guideline in relation to your specialty.', and 'What do you understand by the Hospital at Night (H@N) scheme?' See Chapter 10 for more information on management.

Clinical experience

The aim of this part of the interview is to determine your suitability for entry at ST level. The interviewers will have a copy of your application form, and as an opening question you might be asked to discuss your clinical experience to date. In these types of question, the interviewer does not want to hear a list of hospitals and dates of when you worked there. Instead, you need to relate your personal story, and you may be asked to discuss one or two jobs in more critical detail. One approach would be to discuss all the positive things that you have gained out of each of your posts. If a particular post was somewhat weak in one area you should acknowledge this, but also explain how you addressed the situation; for example: 'My exposure to X was poor in this post, but in my next job there was more than ample opportunity to remedy this deficiency in my training.' This makes it appear that you are planning your career sensibly.

Other questions in this section will often be related to clinical scenarios. There are a huge number of clinical scenarios that can arise and they will depend on which specialty you are applying to. Most scenarios are based on real incidents, so the interviewers will be looking for evidence that you are safe, and whether you have had hands-on experience or the skills necessary to cope with your level of entry into specialist training. Moreover, are you going to be a coherent, sensible voice at the end of the phone at 2am?

Often the scenarios will relate to the management of a medical or surgical emergency, such as an acute exacerbation of asthma, a massive GI bleed or a trauma patient brought into 'resus'. Alternatively, scenarios may be based around cases commonly encountered in either an accident and emergency or outpatient setting; examples are the management of an elderly patient with iron-deficiency anaemia, or an 85-year-old diabetic with a 5-day history of vomiting and abdominal pain. Other scenarios may relate to practical procedures, such as insertion of a central venous pressure catheter, or even male catheterisation. In the weeks before the interview you should prepare by going through clinical cases that you have seen or ones you believe may be important to the specialty you are applying to.

At interview, you need to listen carefully to the clinical scenario, as the wording will often give you clues as to what the interviewer is trying to probe from you. With clinical scenarios, although there is often more than one way to manage the case, the fundamentals will remain the same. Management means resuscitation, taking a history, examining the patient, formulating a differential diagnosis, investigating the patient, establishing a definitive diagnosis, and giving treatment. Importantly, you should also demonstrate a multidisciplinary approach to the patient's care involving other specialists (e.g. radiologists, neurosurgeons, anaesthetists) and your seniors/consultant as appropriate. You should not be afraid to ask for help.

Throughout this station you should demonstrate a logical approach and demonstrate a clear understanding of the management of the condition in your answer. If you really don't know, rather than make things up, you should say you don't know, but would seek advice from a senior colleague. Also, if you forget something important in a patient's management, you should acknowledge this. Don't leave long silences while you try to think of your next step; it is much better to say that you have forgotten or that you do not know and to move on to the next topic. It will usually be quite apparent to the panel members that this is just a short memory lapse.

Other questions in this station may be designed to test a combination of qualities as defined in the person specification. For example: 'You have two patients presenting in A&E at the same time, one with a suspected ruptured abdominal aortic aneurysm, a second with a gastric perforation. Your FY1 is concerned about an unwell patient on the ward. How would you tackle the situation?' This requires you to demonstrate good communication skills, team-working and leadership, as well as the ability to keep calm under pressure, and rapidly assess, prioritise and recognise sick patients. Note that in these scenarios you are not expected to be in more than one place at the same time. However, by using effective communication and calling for help early, as well as delegating tasks, this scenario may be managed successfully with no detrimental effect on patient care.

Behavioural questions

Other qualities in the person specification may be assessed using situational or behavioural questions in addition to, or as part of, more generic questions.

Work-related behavioural or situational questions are becoming increasingly more popular in medicine and are used to assess your performance in the past – the reasoning being that past performance is often the best predictor of future performance in a similar situation. Situational questions are thought to be more objective than traditional questions; so, following an often very open-ended starting question, the interviewer can then probe deeper with further questions, such as 'How did you feel at the time?'

Although there are a vast number of potential situational questions, it is useful to think of a handful of scenarios beforehand that can be adapted to cover the most common questions or which demonstrate the necessary key person-specific qualities. Each answer should be specific and incorporate some background/scene-setting information (this should be brief), the specific action you took (which demonstrates a specific quality within the person specification) and the positive outcome. An example of a situational question is: 'Describe a time when you have had to coordinate the activities of a team in a critical situation and how you dealt with the stress.' This question assesses both your ability to cope with stress as well as manage others within a team and problem-solve. You should use 'real' examples in your response, and avoid embellishing the truth.

Other so-called generic questions may more specifically target one aspect of the person specification. For example, to assess your 'vigilance and situational awareness' you may be asked: 'Describe an example from your experience in this specialty when applying your clinical judgement had a defining impact on patient management. What did you do and how do you think the outcome was affected by your judgement?'. To assess your ability to teamwork, you may be asked: 'How do you ensure good teamwork?', ' What is a team and why is teamwork important?', or 'Give an example where you showed leadership'. Although, at a junior doctor level, you are not expected to have developed the same level of leadership skills as your more senior colleagues, applicants should be able to demonstrate a clear understanding of the attributes that make a good leader and be seen to be starting to develop these skills.

To assess your 'problem solving and decision making' you could be asked: 'How do you deal with a patient who presents with a condition that you are unfamiliar with?'. To assess your 'organisation and planning' skills you could be asked: 'How do you effectively organise your day?' ... and so forth.

Difficult interview questions

Difficult interview questions often draw on multiple aspects of the person specification. Good examples are those relating to conflict at work. This could be a conflict with a colleague (e.g. a senior doctor who refuses to review a sick patient), another healthcare professional (e.g. a nurse who disagrees with your management plan), or a relative who is unhappy with a family member's care and is rather aggressive. Conflict-type questions are common and need careful preparation, but your answer will inevitably involve communication skills, negotiation and initiative, empathy, team-working, and possibly also clinical incidence reporting. You must emphasise that you would listen to the views of all involved in the altercation, and then negotiate some form of mutually acceptable resolution.

Another difficult question may centre on colleagues in unusual situations. For example: 'How do you manage a colleague who is working under the influence of alcohol or drugs?' Importantly, you should remember that you have a duty of care to your patient. *Good Medical Practice* clearly states:

> You must protect patients from risk of harm posed by another colleague's conduct, performance or health. The safety of patients must come first at all times. If you have concerns that a colleague may not be fit to practise, you must take appropriate steps without delay, so that the concerns are investigated and patients protected where necessary.

It is important to appreciate that 'difficult' doctors may themselves be in difficulty. They could be under work pressure (conflict with colleagues/ managers) or personal pressure (domestic, financial, bereavement), or be ill, or not coping (physically or mentally), be insecure, be inadequately trained, lack motivation etc. There are a number of avenues available to you to resolve this dilemma. Local systems should be in place, and you should initially attempt to seek local resolution. If you feel you can, it may be appropriate to talk to the doctor involved directly. If not, you should contact an appropriate lead within your Trust, such as the clinical director, educational supervisor, senior clinician or deanery. Where local mechanisms fail, you should consider contacting the General Medical Council.

Communication skills

Your communication skills will be continuously assessed throughout the course of the interview, so you should be aware of your body-language and language use throughout the day.

Communication skills can also be more formally assessed within a communications station. This may use role playing with the use of actors/ patients or the interviewer. Common scenarios encountered include:

- consent for a procedure such as a colonoscopy
- breaking bad news, for example to a patient with cancer
- dealing with difficult patients, such as a patient who refuses treatment and wishes to self-discharge

- dealing with difficult colleagues
- a telephone call to your consultant, perhaps to discuss patients admitted on call.

Good communication (i.e. listening, negotiation and compromise to reach a resolution) is usually the mainstay in management of these scenarios (Box 2.4).

The General Medical Council's document *Good Medical Practice* (2006) gives guidelines on effectively communicating with patients:

- Listen to your patients.
- Ask for and respect their views.
- Respond to their concerns and preferences.
- Share with patients, in a way they can understand, the information they want or need to know about their condition, its likely progression, and the treatment options available to them, including associated risks and uncertainties.
- Respond to patients' questions and keep them informed about the progress of their care.
- Make sure that patients are informed about how information is shared within teams and among those who will be providing their care.
- Make sure, wherever practicable, that arrangements are made to meet patients' language and communication needs.

Box 2.4 GMC guidelines for effective communication

Finally, be aware that there have been more novel methods used to assess your ability to communicate, so you should not be too surprised if you are asked to describe a random set of items on a table.

Presentations

Communication may be assessed at interview by asking you to give a presentation, either unplanned or pre-planned. Some interviews will merely assess the content of presentations but others will mark the content as well.

If pre-planned, you will usually be advised of the topic of the presentation at the time of notification of the interview. The possible topics are varied and can be medical/clinical (where the emphasis is often on audit, medical ethics or the multidisciplinary approach to patient care) or non-medical, where the emphasis is often on topics such as team building, management, problem solving and communication skills.

All the shortlisted candidates will be given the same topic, so the panel could have heard the same or similar points being made several times by the time you are seen. Try to make your presentation unique and sound enthusiastic. Finally, keep to time as you may be cut short if you don't. Box 2.5 has some tips for a pre-planned presentation.

- Your presentation should be in Microsoft PowerPoint and in landscape.
- The first slide should contain the presentation title and your name only.
- Do not overcrowd your slides. Ideally there should be no more than four or five bullet points or 9–15 words per slide.
- As a rule of thumb, you should expect to take 30–40 seconds per slide (may be up to 2 minutes for more complex slides) and you should adjust your total number of slides to your time limit.
- Choose the size of the font carefully – ideally it should be size 28 or greater.
- Avoid using a busy or distracting background. Stick to a plain or non-offensive slide background.
- Choose the text and background colours carefully. Try to avoid reds and greens as an interviewer might be colour-blind.
- Avoid excess animation. Focus on the content of your presentation; now is not the time to work on getting laughs.
- Don't simply read your slides. The bullets on the slides should merely be a prompt and summary of the salient points. Keep this simple.
- Speak clearly and confidently and make eye-contact with the interviewers.
- Pace the presentation. Don't suddenly realise in the last 30 seconds that you still have a third of the presentation left to go through.
- Practise your presentation, if possible in front of friends or colleagues who can suggest ways to improve it as well as ask questions.
- Make sure that you keep to the time allowed.
- When delivering your presentation, watch where you stand and ensure you don't obscure or detract attention from your slides.
- If you are likely to need a laser-pointer, take one with you.
- Draw up a list of possible questions you might be asked and be prepared with answers.
- When answering questions, don't be defensive or argumentative.
- Take a back-up copy, perhaps on a different memory stick or email yourself an extra copy.

Box 2.5 General tips on preparing a presentation

Alternatively, you may be asked just 20–30 minutes before the interview to prepare a 2- or 3-minute presentation. You might be allowed to use a visual aid, usually an acetate or poster board. The topics are likely to be generic, such as: 'Why are you the best person for the job?', 'Why have you chosen this specialty?', or 'Describe your strengths and weaknesses.' The purpose of this second type of presentation, in addition to assessing your communication and presentation skills, is to assess your ability to think 'on your feet', manage your time effectively, and be dynamic.

When you are given only a short time to prepare a presentation, the same general principles apply. However, under these circumstances the interviewers will expect you to be a bit nervous, so don't worry if you stutter or the presentation doesn't go quite to plan.

Practical skills

There might be a station designed specifically to assess your practical ability. This station is more likely to be present in the craft specialties and will, generally speaking, involve quite simple tasks such as suturing and tying knots. Some skills may require familiarity with commonly used instruments in that specialty. For instance, in otolaryngology, familiarity with microscopes would be an important practical skill. Cardiopulmonary resuscitation (CPR) stations are increasingly popular for some specialties.

Critical analysis

Candidates may be asked to critically appraise (read, interpret and summarise) a medical or even a non-medical paper prior to the interview and asked to either present or discuss the paper at interview. The time allowed to prepare can vary from 20 to 40 minutes, following which you may be asked to either present the paper or be asked questions on it. This may include assessment of your understanding of research statistics (e.g. linear regression analysis), or research ethics and principles. Attending a journal club is a good way to prepare for this type of interview.

Group discussion

Group discussion stations are aimed at assessing how you interact with others (engage, communicate, influence) and not necessarily your clinical knowledge or skills, although the group task may require an understanding of your specialty and the structure of the NHS. The interviewer may form part of the group or be an observer. The group will usually consist of 4–6 people, and you may be asked to complete a task or find a solution to a difficult case or solve an ethical dilemma.

After the interview

When you go to the interview, check that the recruiting office has your correct contact details should you be made an offer, and also advise the office of any reason or period of time when you might not be contactable.

Receiving offers

Offers of posts to training programmes will be made (usually by email or even text message) to interviewees who are ranked the highest at interview. When an offer is made you will have a limited time to accept or decline it, after which the offer will be withdrawn. Unlike in previous years, offers for first-round posts will be made at the same time (at the beginning of March). If this is the best offer on the table, you should accept it as soon as possible, and it is wise to telephone your deanery to ensure they have received your email of acceptance. At the same time you should decline any other offers you may also have, as these can be offered to other applicants. If you have accepted a job offer previously, it may be possible to upgrade your offer (see Chapter 1). If you don't have any other offers on the table, you need to think carefully before declining an offer.

Once you have accepted a training programme, the deanery will match you to a specific post/rotation within the programme, and should advise you of the following:

● the name of your employer
● the start date and length (or likely length) of the period of employment
● the name of the position to be filled and the work to be done
● the location of the work and the hours to be worked
● possible health and safety risks
● the qualifications/experience required to do the job
● expenses payable (e.g. removal/relocation)
● the minimum rate of remuneration payable and any other benefits on offer, and the intervals at which you will be paid
● the notice period.

There will be the usual employment checks, including verification of references, fitness-to-practice updates from the GMC, occupational health clearance, Criminal Records Bureau (CRB) disclosures and immigration status checks, as a minimum. When these checks have been successfully completed, your new employer will confirm the post and you should receive your contract within two months of starting in post.

What if I'm not offered the post?

You will be contacted by email if you are unsuccessful at interview. You can contact (write or email) your recruiting office to request feedback about your performance and to seek careers advice. If you do this, you should ask for your rank and/or score, the rank/score required to receive an offer, and the total number of applicants interviewed by the deanery. You can also request copies of your interview score sheets. This information can guide your preparation for future interviews. In addition, you should reconsider whether the specialty/deanery you have chosen is realistic.

Finally, you may still have a shot at the post you want, as deaneries will continue to advertise training vacancies beyond the first and second rounds throughout the year as they arise.

Sources of further information

Academic posts: www.nihrtcc.nhs.uk

GP training: http://gprecruitment.oth.uk

Postgraduate Medical Education and Training Board (PMETB): www.pmetb.org.uk

Recruitment to medical specialty training in Northern Ireland: www.nimdta.gov.uk

Recruitment to medical specialty training in Scotland: www.mmc.scot.nhs.uk

Recruitment to medical specialty training in Wales: www.mmcwales.org

3

Specialist examinations

Key aims of this chapter

- Explain why specialist exams exist
- Give an overview of exit or specialist exams in the various areas of medicine
- Discuss when to sit them and how to apply.

Introduction

Medicine can sometimes seem like one long exam. Through medical school, foundation and core training you are bombarded by exams and assessments. Your exit or subspecialty exam is another such hurdle, but with it comes a certain amount of excitement – as it brings you in sight of the light at the end of the tunnel and your final destination. Moreover, certainly at the time of writing, it will be the final exam of your career (not regarding revalidation).

Exit and specialty examinations

Exit exams are knowledge-based and are undertaken in the last few years of training. Success in these is a requirement for completion of specialist training and acceptance on to the specialist register (although it does not guarantee this). The purpose of these forms of assessment is to ensure that certified specialists have sufficient knowledge in their specialty to become competent consultants. In addition, they serve to reassure the public of standards in medicine and as a gauge against which physicians working outside the UK can measure their level of attainment.

Which specialties have exit or subspecialty exams?

Exams will vary in format according to your specialty. Indeed, some specialties do not yet have any specialty exam. The aim of this chapter is to discuss the various specialty exams, the best time to take them, and how to go about applying.

Surgery

Subspecialty examinations resulting in the award of a Fellowship of the Royal College of Surgeons (FRCS) have been in existence for decades. The original fellowship was available in general surgery and the subspecialties of ophthalmic surgery, ENT surgery, and obstetrics and gynaecology. Exams now extend to include several other subspecialties including orthopaedics, urology and maxillofacial surgery (Table 3.1).

Following success in the exam, a suffix denoting the subspecialty is applied to the FRCS title; for example, FRCS (Gen Surg) for general surgery and FRCS (Urol) for urology. In order to use these letters after your name, you will need to maintain payment of your fellowship fees to your affiliated or allocated royal college.

How do I apply to sit the exam?

The Joint Committee on Intercollegiate Examinations (JCIE) is responsible for overseeing the surgical specialty examinations for the nine intercollegiate boards (listed in Table 3.1) and reports to the four surgical Royal Colleges of UK and Ireland.

In order to be eligible to apply, applicants must:

- hold a medical degree recognised for registration by the General Medical Council of the United Kingdom or the Medical Council of Ireland
- have maintained payment of their affiliated or designated college subscription fees, following success in the MRCS exams
- provide evidence of having reached the required standard of clinical competence defined in the Intercollegiate Surgical Curriculum – this evidence consists of three structured references, your CV and logbook.

Application to sit the FRCS examination is made via the Intercollegiate Specialty Board (ISB) online application system, and the exam currently carries a fee of £1795 (£520 for Section 1 and £1275 for Section 2). These fees unfortunately cannot be claimed against personal tax.

Table 3.1: Details of specialty examinations in surgery

Specialty	Suffix	Exam parts	Eligibility	Frequency
Cardiothoracic surgery	C-Th	**Section 1** (written) Paper 1 – SBAs (2 hours) Paper 2 – EMIs (2.5 hours) **Section 2** (oral) A series of structured interviews: a Cardiac surgery long case (30 mins) b Thoracic surgery long case (30 mins) c Cardiac surgery short case (30 mins) d Thoracic surgery short case (30 mins) e Cardiac surgery viva (30 mins) f Thoracic surgery viva (30 mins)	● Min 6 years post qualification ● Evidence of appropriate competency level ● Eligibility for registration with GMC	Section 1 Twice yearly (Jan/July) Section 2 Twice yearly (May/Oct)
General surgery	Gen Surg	**Section 1** (written) Paper 1 – SBAs (2 hours) Paper 2 – EMIs (2.5 hours) **Section 2** (clinical and oral) *Clinical exam* with two sessions of short cases, each lasting for 30 mins (one of these may be in your declared subspecialty, if given) *Oral exam* which is composed of three vivas in the following areas: ● Emergency surgery with critical care (30 mins) ● General surgery and subspecialty (30 mins) ● Academic (20 mins) where you will be given two papers to read and prepare over the course of an hour and then examined for 10 mins on each paper	● Evidence of appropriate competency level ● Eligibility for registration with GMC ● Maintenance of affiliated or allocated college fees	Section 1 Thrice yearly (Feb/June/Nov) Section 2 Thrice yearly (Feb/May-June/Sept)

(Continued)

Table 3.1: (*Continued*)

Specialty	Suffix	Exam parts	Eligibility	Frequency
Neurosurgery	Neuro Surg	**Section 1** (written) Paper 1 – SBAs (2 hours) Paper 2 – EMIs (2.5 hours) **Section 2** (clinical and oral) Scenario-based and patient-based cases and divided into: *Long case* (approx 10 mins for history and presentation of salient points, 10 mins for examination, differential diagnosis and investigation, and 10 mins for a discussion of a management plan, treatment options, and potential complications (30 mins in total) *Short cases* testing clinical knowledge, diagnostic acumen, investigations and interpretation, treatment options and taking consent *Three vivas:* ● Operative surgery and surgical anatomy (30 mins) ● Investigation of the neurosurgical patient, including neuroradiology (30 mins) ● Non-operative clinical practice of neurosurgery (30 mins)	● Min 6 years post qualification ● Evidence of appropriate competency level ● Eligibility for registration with GMC	Section 1 Twice yearly (Jan/July) Section 2 Twice yearly (March/Oct)
Oral and maxillofacial surgery	OMFS	**Section 1** (written) Paper 1 – SBAs (2 hours) Paper 2 – EMIs (2.5 hours) **Section 2** (clinical and oral) One new-patient case (30 mins) Follow-up cases (30 mins)	● Min 5 years post qualification ● Evidence of appropriate competency level ● Eligibility for registration with GMC	Section 1 Twice yearly (Jan/June) Section 2 Twice yearly (March/Sept)

		Three 30-min *oral* exams covering topics from sections A, B and C below: ● Section A: aesthetic surgery; craniofacial surgery; cleft lip and palate orthognathic surgery ● Section B: head and neck oncology; head and neck reconstruction; oral medicine and pathology; salivary gland surgery and pathology; surgical dermatology ● Section C: dentoalveolar surgery/implantology; maxillofacial trauma; orofacial infections and emergency surgery; orofacial pain/TMJ		
Otolaryngology	ORL-HNS	**Section 1** (written) Paper 1 – SBAs (2 hours) Paper 2 – EMIs (2.5 hours) **Section 2** (oral and practical) Four oral exams in: ● Otology including neuro-otology (30 mins) ● Head and neck surgery (30 mins) ● Paediatric otolaryngology (30 mins) ● Rhinology and facial plastics (30 mins) (Facial plastics will cover otoplasty, rhinoplasty, flap reconstruction, excision of facial lesions, suturing techniques, tissue handling and assessment of patients undergoing cosmetic procedures) (30 mins) *Practical* exam in operative surgery (20-min session) involving temporal bone dissection +/– cadaveric head and neck specimens, endoscopic examination of the cadaveric nose	● Min 6 years post qualification ● Evidence of appropriate competency level ● Eligibility for registration with GMC	Section 1 Twice yearly (Jan/July) Section 2 Twice yearly (Apr/Nov)

Table 3.1: *(Continued)*

Specialty	Suffix	Exam parts	Eligibility	Frequency
Paediatric surgery	Paed Surg	**Section 1** (written) Paper 1 – SBAs (2 hours) Paper 2 – EMIs (2.5 hours) **Section 2** (oral) Three structured interview scenarios: ● Urology and neonatal urology (40 mins) ● Oncology and endocrine neonatal surgery (40 mins) ● General and gastrointestinal surgery, emergency surgery and trauma	● Min 6 years post qualification ● Evidence of appropriate competency level ● Eligibility for registration with GMC	Section 1 Twice yearly (June/Nov) Section 2 Twice yearly (March/Sept)
Plastic surgery	Plast	**Section 1** (written) Paper 1 – SBAs (2 hours) Paper 2 – EMIs (2.5 hours) **Section 2** (clinical and oral) Medium/long cases (30 mins) in which two patients will be seen Two short cases (30 mins each) in which five patients will be seen Oral exam is in the following areas: ● Trauma/burns (30 mins) ● Acute head and neck tumours; initial cleft management; genitourinary (30 mins) ● Basic sciences and generic/aesthetic/ethics/consent issues (30 mins)	● Min 6 years post qualification ● Evidence of appropriate competency level ● Eligibility for registration with GMC	Section 1 Twice yearly (June/Nov) Section 2 Twice yearly (March/Sept)

| Trauma and orthopaedics | Tr and Orth | **Section 1** (written)
Paper 1 – SBAs (2 hours + extra 15 mins for reading time for the published paper – the first 12 questions of this paper will relate to this)
Paper 2 – EMIs (2.5 hours)
Section 2 (clinical and vivas)
Two sessions of clinical intermediate cases (15 mins each)
Two sessions of clinical short cases (15 mins each on upper limb and lower limb)
Vivas in the following areas:
● Adult elective orthopaedics including spine (30 mins)
● Trauma including spine (30 mins)
● Children's orthopaedics / hand and upper limb (30 mins)
● Applied basic sciences related to orthopaedics | ● Min 6 years post qualification
● Evidence of appropriate competency level
● Eligibility for registration with GMC | Section 1
Thrice yearly (Feb/ June/Nov)
Section 2
Thrice yearly (Feb/ Apr/Nov) |
| Urology | Urol | **Section 1** (written)
Paper 1 – SBAs (2 hours)
Paper 2 – EMIs (2.5 hours)
Section 2 (clinical)
Eight 20-min clinical scenarios in the following areas:
● Session 1: urological oncology (kidney and bladder); urological oncology (prostate, testis and penis)
● Session 2: paediatric urology; emergency urology
● Session 3: calculi and urinary tract infections; urological imaging and principles of urological technology
● Session 4: bladder dysfunction; gynaecological aspects of urology BPH and andrology | ● Min 6 years post qualification
● Evidence of appropriate competency level
● Eligibility for registration with GMC | Section 1
Twice yearly (Jan/ July)
Section 2
Twice yearly (May/ Nov) |

When should I sit the exam?

The FRCS is an expensive examination, so unless you want to go down the path of remortgaging your house or selling off the household silver, start revision early and be prepared. The recommendation is to take the exam when you have the necessary amount of clinical expertise behind you, ideally in the penultimate year of training. However, this isn't a rigid requirement and it is not uncommon to see candidates sitting the exam at an earlier time. There are no rules as to when to start revising, and most people start some form of revision six months ahead of time; but people vary in their revision styles, and by now in your career you will have a technique that works for you.

What is the format of the exam?

The examination for the FRCS is mapped according to the curriculum available for each specialty. These are available at www.iscp.ac.uk.

The format for the FRCS is similar across the specialties. In general, the exam consists of two parts, a written and a clinical and viva component, and specialties usually differ in the formatting of the clinical component.

The written exam has two papers:

- Paper 1 lasts for 2 hours and is composed of Single Best Answer (SBA) questions.
- Paper 2 lasts for 2.5 hours and is composed of Extended Matching Item (EMI) questions.

Questions are *not* negatively marked, and the mean of both marks will determine your overall score and thus eligibility to proceed to Section 2 of the exam.

Section 1 has, since January 2011, been delivered via computer-based testing (CBT) and can be undertaken at any one of 150 or more Pearson VUE professional test centres in the UK and Ireland, and Section 2 at a designated centre – typically a hospital.

Section 2 of the FRCS exam is the clinical component and assesses knowledge of anatomy, physiology and pathology through a series of vivas and clinical scenarios. The clinical component for the various surgical specialties are outlined in Table 3.1.

How should I prepare for the exam?

The FRCS exam sets questions that are very clinical (which surprises many people) and these very much aim to assess your approach to the management of a patient. Revision therefore also needs to take this approach. For example, in Sections 1 and 2, although an appreciation of the basic sciences is necessary, you are unlikely (in contrast to the MRCS exams) to be asked purely anatomy-based questions, and more likely to be asked – in the FRCS (General Surgery) – about the adverse drug reactions related to for example, common immunosuppressive agents used in renal transplantation, or to calculate the Nottingham score in a number of given clinical scenarios. Sample questions are available at www. intercollegiate.org.uk, and revision websites, courses and texts exist.

Medicine

The MRCP(UK) examination, consisting of Parts 1, Part 2 Written and Part 2 Clinical (PACES), is the main knowledge-based examination for medical trainees in their early part of training, and a mandatory requirement for ST3 entry into the medical specialties. Moreover, candidates who entered CMT after August 2009 cannot exit from their programme until they have successfully achieved all components of the MRCP(UK) exam.

Subspecialty examinations are a relatively new phenomenon in medicine and are now compulsory for achieving CCT for all UK trainees who commenced specialist training in or after August 2007 (for those commencing specialty training before this date the specialty exam is optional). The Specialty Certificate Examinations (SCEs) were established in response to PMETB's requirement to include an assessment of knowledge in higher specialty training. In 2006, the first pilot of the Specialty Certificate Examination took place and SCEs have now been rolled out across the following specialties:

- acute internal medicine – with the exception of those on the 2007 GIM (Acute) curriculum, which leads to a CCT in general internal medicine which does not attract an SCE
- dermatology
- endocrinology and diabetes
- gastroenterology
- geriatric medicine
- infectious diseases
- medical oncology
- nephrology
- neurology
- palliative medicine
- respiratory medicine
- rheumatology.

Success in the SCE results in the award of a certificate. In addition, UK trainees with the MRCP(UK) who pass the SCE in their specialty and who are recommended for a CCT are granted the post-nominal MRCP(UK) (Specialty).

There are a number of specialties that accept entry into specialty training from routes other than CMT (Table 3.2). These trainees will therefore not possess the MRCP(UK), and, provided trainees from these routes fulfil the requirements for these alternative pathways, they will continue on to a CCT programme.

When should I sit the exam?

You can take the SCE in your specialty onwards of ST4 (the second year of specialty training) and you should attempt the exam at least once by the time you reach your penultimate year and at least twice before your proposed CCT date. Importantly, there is no limit on the number of times you can take the exam; however, it will affect your eligibility for, and prolong the date to, your CCT (although the latter will be at the discretion of your postgraduate dean).

Table 3.2: Pathways (source: www.rcp.london.ac.uk)

Specialty	Alternative entry pathways
Audiological medicine	MRCPCH, MRCS, MRCGP
Clinical genetics	MRCPCH
Clinical neurophysiology	MRCPCH
Dermatology	MRCPCH
Haematology	MRCPCH
Palliative medicine	MRCPCH, MRCS, FRCA
Medical ophthalmology	Can enter via surgical ophthalmology but must achieve MRCP(UK)
Nuclear medicine	FRCR
Paediatric cardiology	MRCPCH
Pharmaceutical medicine	Can enter from any clinical specialty but must have the relevant equivalent of MRCP(UK)
Rehabilitation medicine	MRCS, MRCPsych, MRCGP
Sport and exercise medicine	MRCGP

How do I apply to sit the exam?

Application is made via an online system (at My MRCP(UK)), where you are also able to pay the fee, track the status of your application, select your test centre (through Pearson Vue) and review results – which are usually available four weeks after the exam.

If you undertook the SCEs in 2008, 2009 or 2010, there is a one-off fee of £800 for the exam, which allows for up to two sittings of the exam. From 2011, the fee is for one sitting only, and exams currently are run only once a year. This perhaps makes the case for sitting the exam early.

What is the format of the exam?

The SCEs have been developed by the Royal College of Physicians (RCP) in conjunction with the MRCP(UK) Examinations Department and the specialist societies. Their focus is on the knowledge required of a newly appointed consultant, and this is the same approach you should take when revising.

Each is composed of two 3-hour SBA papers each containing 100 predominantly scenario-based questions, with an emphasis on diagnosis, investigation, management and prognosis of patients. It is delivered in a computer-based format: questions are delivered electronically and answers recorded electronically, at your selected test centre (run by Pearson VUE). The exam is positively marked.

Radiology

To be eligible to enter the Fellow of the Royal College of Radiologists (FRCR) examination you need to be in a recognised radiology training post. The exam is in two parts, the First and the Final.

The First Part of the FRCR

This is held three times a year and comprises two modules in physics and radiological anatomy (previously just one module in physics). There is no option to compensate in this exam, so you need to pass each part independently.

● The physics module consists of a 2-hour paper-based exam. There are 40 multiple-choice questions (MCQs). These questions are positively marked.

- The anatomy module is examined by a 75-minute image-viewing session consisting of 20 cases/images each followed by five questions. Cases are presented digitally using workstations and Osirix software.

The Final Part of the FRCR

This is held twice a year and has two parts.

Part A, usually held in March and September, examines the basic sciences (physics, anatomy and techniques) over six modules. In order to sit this exam you need to be in a radiology training post and have completed the first part of the FRCR exam.

Each module has one 2-hour paper containing 75 single best answer (SBA) questions. Questions are positively marked. The six modules are:

1   Cardiothoracic and Vascular
2   Musculoskeletal and Trauma
3   Gastrointestinal
4   Genitourinary, Adrenal, Obstetrics and Gynaecology, and Breast
5   Paediatric
6   Central Nervous and Head/Neck.

Part B is usually held twice a year, in April and October. In order to sit this section you should have successfully completed all modules of Part A and completed 2.5 years of radiology training. The exam has three components:

- a reporting session (1 hour) during which you are asked to report on six cases (these may be on CT, US, radionuclide or MR imaging)
- a rapid reporting session (35 minutes) during which you are asked to review a set of 30 cases (a mixture of normal and abnormal)
- an oral session during which you are asked to report on and discuss a number of cases presented on hard-copy film.

Application to the exam

Application to the FRCR is made through the Royal College of Radiologists. Applications typically close 4–6 weeks before the proposed exam dates.

Pathology

Fellowship of the Royal College of Pathologists (FRCPath) is achieved as a trainee by examination. As with other specialty exams, success indicates that you have reached the required standard for independent practice and, as a UK trainee, fulfilled an entry requirement for the Certificate of Eligibility for Specialist Registration (CESR) and entry to the Specialist Register.

Am I eligible to sit the exam?

To be eligible you need first to fulfill the recommended training requirements – for Part 1, at least one year in specialty training, and for Part 2 at least two years in specialty training. You must also be deemed ready to sit the exam by your educational supervisor. In addition, you should be registered and have a primary medical or dental qualification approved by the GMC or General Dental Council (GDC). Notably with respect to eligibility, forensic pathology, histopathology, neuropathology and paediatric pathology are open only to medical candidates; and oral pathology is open only to dental candidates. Exams are held for most specialties on a twice-yearly basis (there are a number of exceptions).

Success in the Part 1 written paper is a requirement to progress to Part 2, and on completion of Part 1 you will be offered Associate status in your chosen specialty.

You can sit Part 1 up to four times but only under exceptional circumstances will you be allowed further attempts. You can sit Part 2 *only* in the same subject as Part 1, unless you seek specific prior permission, or have passed the Part 1 in histopathology when then you could sit the Part 2 in either forensic pathology, neuropathology or paediatric pathology.

The FRCPath exam

This is a knowledge-based test and consists of two parts.

Part 1, depending on your specialty in pathology, consists of either MCQs or EMQs, or short answer and essay papers. For essay papers there is a 'closed' marking system whereby each question is allocated 25 marks, and papers are marked with an Excellent pass, Clear pass, Pass, Borderline fail, Clear fail or Bad fail. There is the opportunity to compensate by performing better on another paper. For short-answer papers, marks are allocated separately for each question and the pass mark for each paper will vary. MCQ/EMQ exams, where applicable, are 3 hours in length and are not negatively marked.

Part 2 is a practical exam and may also involve a project, depending on your subspecialty.

Application to the exam

Application for each examination date is by submission of the printed application form to the Examinations Department at www.rcpath.org/exams.

Anaesthetics

Fellowship of the Royal College of Anaesthetists (FRCA) is achieved by examination in two parts, the Primary and the Final.

Am I eligible to sit the exam?

You are eligible to take the FRCA if you hold a UK training post or have held a UK training post in anaesthetics in the past five years. Staff and associate specialist (SAS) doctors are exempt from the five-year rule. In September 2011, the criteria for eligibility for the Primary FRCA was extended to be more inclusive of non-UK trainees, and by September 2012 it will extend to all components of the FRCA. Importantly, success in the primary FRCA is a requirement for entry into ST3.

The Primary FRCA

This is divided into two parts.

- A 3-hour MCQ paper contains 60 multiple false/true (MTF) questions and 30 SBAs on the topics of pharmacology, physiology and physics. The exam is positively marked, with one mark given for a correct answer in the MTF section and four marks given for each correct SBA question. You can sit this exam a maximum of five times.
- The clinical part is as follows (a maximum of four attempts may be made):
  - an 'objective' structured clinical examination (1 hour 50 mins), with 18 stations (16 of which count) in resuscitation, technical skills, anatomy (general procedures), history-taking, physical examination, communication skills, anaesthetic equipment, monitoring equipment, measuring equipment, anaesthetic hazards, and the interpretation of X-rays
  - a structured oral exam (SOEs) consisting of three questions on pharmacology and three questions on physiology and biochemistry (30 mins total)
  - a second structured oral exam consisting of three questions on physics, clinical measurement equipment and safety, and three questions on clinical topics (30 mins total).

The Final FRCA

To be eligible for this part you need to have been successful in the Primary exam and be in anaesthetic practice for a minimum of 12 months prior to the date of the exam (there are exceptions to this). The exam itself is again divided into two sections, the written and the SOE.

- The written part can be taken a maximum of six times.
  - The MCQ papor (3 hours) contains 60 MTF and SBA questions covering medicine and surgery, applied basic science, intensive care medicine, pain management and clinical anaesthesia. This exam is positively marked.
  - The SAQ paper (3 hours) contains 12 compulsory questions on the principles and practice of clinical anaesthesia.
- The structured oral exam can be attempted up to six times. It comprises of two vivas, on the topics of:
  - clinical anaesthesia (50 mins)
  - clinical science (30 mins).

Application to the exam

More information and guidance on application to the FRCA can be found at www.rcoa.ac.uk.

Psychiatry

For Membership of the Royal College of Psychiatrists you will need to have 24 months' post-foundation/internship experience in psychiatry and have passed all components of the MRCPsych examination. The exam has two parts (three written papers and a clinical component).

Am I eligible to sit this exam?

You are eligible if you are registered with the GMC and have 6 months' post-foundation experience in an approved training programme or post recognised by the Trust as incorporating educational training (this does not include Trust grade or pilot ST posts).

There is currently no restriction on the number of times you can sit the exam. However, you have 1643 days from the date of achieving a pass in the first written paper taken (1, 2 or 3) to complete all other components of the MRCPsych including the clinical component (the so-called 'Written Paper Validity' period). This period can be extended under exceptional circumstances, such as if you have taken time out for pregnancy or research, or are on a flexible training programme. Failure to achieve all parts within the given time frame means re-sitting all of the written components.

The written papers

Papers 1, 2 and 3 are each 3 hours long and contain 200 questions. Each paper contains a combination of SBA and EMI questions (EMIs form approximately a third of the paper).

The clinical component

This is called the Clinical Assessment of Skills and Competencies (CASC). To be eligible to take this part you must have the support of a sponsor and have:

- completed 24 months of whole-time-equivalent posts in psychiatry (posts must be of either 4 or 6 months duration, and a minimum of 12 months should be spent in general adult psychiatry)
- successfully completed Papers 1, 2 and 3 or passed Part 1 and Paper 3 of the MRCPsych.

You can sit the CASC up to three times, after which you will require a letter of support from your college tutor (or equivalent) requesting any further attempts.

Application to the exam

More information regarding application to the exam can be found at www. rcpsych.ac.uk.

Paediatrics

The examination for Membership of the Royal College of Paediatrics and Child Health (MRCPCH) consists of three sections: Part 1, Part 2 and Clinical. It is an entry requirement for core specialist training in paediatrics. Full information is available from www.rcpch.ac.uk.

Other examinations to consider

The USMLEs

The United States Medical Licensing Examination (USMLE®) is a requirement for medical licensing or practice in the USA. The individual medical licensing authorities ('state medical boards') are responsible for granting a license to practice medicine. Although each medical licensing authority will have its own rules, results of the USMLE form the basis used in granting the initial license to practice medicine.

The USMLE 'assesses a physician's ability to apply knowledge, concepts, and principles, and to demonstrate fundamental patient-centered skills, that are important in health and disease and that constitute the basis of safe and effective patient care'.

Most doctors in the USA will take the USMLEs in medical school, and this or immediately following medical finals is perhaps the best time to take them as a non-American trainee. However, most of us are not that forward-thinking, and leave it until much later. So why take a USMLE? As a specialty trainee in a somewhat uncertain UK medical job market, the USMLEs give you options, both in terms of fellowships in the USA or the option of jumping ship completely.

The exam is divided into three parts or steps. Steps 1 and Step 2-CK (Clinical Knowledge) can be taken at any Prometric test centre worldwide, while Step 2-CS (Clinical Skills) and Step 3 can be taken only in the USA.

Step 1 examines the basic sciences in relation to medical practice and perhaps is the most difficult component of the exam. The subjects covered include anatomy, physiology, biochemistry, pharmacology, pathology, microbiology, genetics and behavioural sciences – so it really is like taking a trip back to preclinical school. It is composed of an 8-hour computer-based exam with 322 MCQs divided over seven blocks, each an hour long, with 46 questions. The pass mark in January 2010 was 188, and the average score 225. If you are considering applying for a residency programme in the USA, your USMLE score for all parts will matter; for a fellowship programme it matters less.

Step 2 is divided into two:

- Step 2-CK assesses your clinical knowledge in medicine, surgery, paediatrics, psychiatry, and obstetrics/gynaecology. It is a 9-hour computer-based assessment with eight blocks each with 44 MCQs.
- Step 2-CS is the clinical component of the exam and is offered in only five centres in the USA.

Step 3 is an assessment which is spread over two days in the USA. On the first day there is an 8-hour computer-based exam with 336 MCQs. On the second day there is a 3-hour computer-based MCQ exam that has 144 questions and nine clinical case simulations.

European specialist examinations

The European Board exams are intended to facilitate movement of specialists between member countries. However, they are not currently an alternative to a national exit or specialist examination, where one exists. Their usefulness is therefore a little dubious, apart from being another addition to your CV.

The exams have two parts. Part 1 is an MCQ paper with 100 questions. Part 2 is the oral or viva component.

There are exams available for a number of medical and surgical specialties, including pathology, neurology, ophthalmology, paediatric surgery, otorhinolaryngology, trauma and orthopaedic surgery, vascular surgery, cardiothoracic surgery, transplant surgery, plastic surgery and dermato-venereology (this is not an exhaustive list).

Sources of further information

Royal College of Anaesthetists: www.rcoa.ac.uk

Royal College of Paediatrics and Child Health: www.rcpch.ac.uk

Royal College of Physicians: www.rcplondon.ac.uk

Royal College of Psychiatrists: www.rcpsych.ac.uk

Royal College of Radiologists: www.rcr.ac.uk

Royal College of Surgeons of England: www.rcseng.ac.uk

USMLE exams: www.usmle.org

4

General practice

Key aims of this chapter

- Important factors to consider as a GP
- Give an overview of life as a GP trainee
- Making the most of your GP training.

Introduction

Many new general practitioners (GPs) feel that the ST3 year is all too brief. It represents a steep learning curve that includes professional examinations, learning on the job in a GP surgery and attempting to pick up some of the business and management skills required for being a GP. This chapter provides a brief heads-up on the environment in which GP ST3s and new practitioners will find themselves. It is easily possible to be so focused on the clinical work and examinations that issues such as preparing for professional life, engaging with professional politics, and opportunities for personal development, can slip you by.

This chapter will look at the primary care setting, the usefulness of key professional bodies to GPs, and making the most of ST3 and the Royal College of General Practitioner's (RCGP) examinations. It then goes on to discuss the types of GP career available and offers an initial approach to interviews for salaried jobs and partnerships. It is intended as a starting point for thinking about ST3 and beyond, so further resources are identified throughout.

ST3 and beyond

A changing and challenging world in primary care

It is worth initially taking a step back to take a brief look at the expectations and challenges for GPs in the UK. In many countries, general practice sits at the heart of healthcare as one of the first points of access for anyone seeking medical care and as the route to specialist or hospital care. In the UK, universal registration with a GP formalises this. There are a number of core features identified with general practice:

- The commitment to the patient, irrespective of his or her state of health, requires a holistic approach to care. These patient-centred techniques are sometimes described as a 'bio-psycho-social' approach.
- The relationship with a patient may take place over a long period. Even where many GPs see the same patient in a practice, there is a continuity of records.
- GPs may have separate or interrelated professional relationships with several members of a family. This may lead to problems with confidentiality or requests to intervene outside of a purely clinical context.
- Surgeries are often close to people's homes so there can be a shared knowledge and understanding of the community. GPs may offer domiciliary care, which many hospital specialties do not. Difficulties in visiting patients at home has been identified as a problem of inner-city general practice.[1]
- This nearness to the community may create an advocacy role for GPs within a community, or a role for the GP to act as the agent of the state in delivering public health messages.
- In the UK, GPs still play a major role in sickness certification.
- In the UK, general practice is still the usual first point of contact for patients seeking medical care. The GP usually acts as a gatekeeper to secondary and tertiary care, and even when this role is not appropriate may assist a patient to choose the best option. It is to the GP that a patient returns when other specialists have concluded their contributions to a patient's care.

So why might it be relevant to think about the GP's role when entering ST3? The RCGP manual for GP-trainers and GP-educators suggests that the following changes in society at large may challenge the GP – patient relationship.[2] Think about how this list and the above relate to your practice as a GP:

- the rise of consumerism in medicine
- an emphasis on patient autonomy

- the changing status of women in society
- the rise of a culture of affirmative action and pride in disability
- attacks on professional self-regulation
- an increasingly litigious environment
- multiculturalism
- social concerns about assault and violence towards women
- holistic and alternative health movements
- the changing status of all professions in society
- a decline of the role of medicine and expansion in the role of other professionals
- increased uses of technology
- a shift of care from hospital to the community
- European working time [regulations]
- increased hospital liability for doctor's care
- administrative – the containment of medical costs
- an increased emphasis on informed consent
- increased attention to prevention, and patient education
- an increasing social acceptance of physician-assisted suicide
- the doctor's role as trustee regarding disability benefits.

*Hint for a SWOT analysis: Have a think about how any of the above list relates to your **S**trengths or **W**eaknesses or represent an **O**pportunity or **T**hreat as a clinician, a potential GP partner, or any other roles you wish to pursue in your career as a GP. You could use this reflection either to enhance your CV, or to identify learning needs for your e-portfolio or appraisal.*

The Royal College of General Practitioners

So why might it be worth considering full membership of the RCGP, beyond the necessary qualification to practise as a GP in the UK?

The RCGP is the academic body for general practice in the UK. It sets academic and clinical standards for the whole profession. It is not a trade union but acts as the voice of the profession on education, training and professional standards. The RCGP is also a good source of accredited continuous professional development (CPD). Like the BMA and the other royal colleges, the RCGP lobbies the government on issues relating to healthcare. Whether through direct involvement in the RCGP, or participation at conferences and consultations, GPs can influence RCGP and (through successful lobbying) government policy. It is relatively straightforward to become involved in the RCGP as a trainee or new practitioner. The RCGP has a federal structure – it is divided into geographical faculties (e.g. there is a North and West London Faculty) which will hold educational meetings and an AGM at which members who want to get involved can approach the faculty board.

This is a great way to meet local GPs in your area or in an area you wish to move to, and a great way to influence CPD availability locally. The RCGP website is a good resource for advice on most matters relating to training and professional development, and includes the RCGP curriculum (see below) which is by definition a benchmark for both trainees and established GPs. The RCGP e-portfolio is an alternative to the NHS appraisal toolkit and is an appropriate tool to record personal development and learning for appraisal and revalidation.

There are two broad types of RCGP membership for fully qualified GPs:[3]

- Associate membership is for trained GPs who do not wish to pursue full membership but wish to retain links with the college. Benefits include receiving the *British Journal of General Practice* and attending educational events, but not the ability to influence RCGP policy.
- Full membership is available to all GPs who have taken the MRCGP examination. Those who qualified before 2007 and did not take MRCGP (which was optional then) may undergo a process called Membership by Assessment of Performance (MAP) to obtain full membership.

The BMA's General Practitioners Committee

In effect, the British Medical Association's GPC is your trade union. It is a committee of the BMA with authority to deal with all matters affecting NHS general practitioners. It is the only body that represents all GPs in Great Britain, whether or not they are members of the BMA, at a national level. The committee is recognised as the sole negotiating body for general practice by the Department of Health and is represented in negotiations with ministers and civil servants by a team of eight GPs elected by the committee.

The GPC is supported in negotiations by expert advisers from the permanent staff of the BMA. The team is supplemented by other GPC members as appropriate, together with legal, accountancy and other specialist advice as and when necessary.

The Welsh and Scottish GPCs are subcommittees of the national GPC but have autonomy on NHS matters exclusive to their countries. The Northern Ireland GPC is autonomous of the GPC, although it has close working relations with it.

Procedures for policy making operate on an annual cycle. Individual GPs can influence policy through their local medical committee (LMC), which considers the annual report and submits motions to the annual conference of LMC representatives in June. This conference, comprising more than 300 GPs, is the principal policy-making body. Its resolutions are referred to the GPC to consider and implement, and in this way the committee represents the interests of GPs as expressed through conference decisions.

So what are the key BMA membership benefits for the individual GP?

- While national representation of GP interests is on behalf of all GPs, individual representation in trade disputes is available to members only. This includes a contract-checking service.
- The BMA's medical ethics department has an advice line – again this is a membership benefit. A brief look at the kinds of advice requested in 2009/10 shows that confidentiality and management of records including the writing of medical reports are a top concern. These are key issues for GPs.[4]
- To get involved (as with the RCGP), one has to be a member. This supports expenses for attending and contributing to the conferences and in turn shaping the environment in which we work.

The ST in ST3 stands for STeep learning curve!

The three-year GP training programme in the UK is one of the shortest training periods for primary care practitioners in Europe. ST3 GP vocational training schemes have a full or half day of education (referred to as day-release, or more flippantly as 'play-school'). These often have a trainee-directed component – if you have identified your learning needs early on, then you can request training in particular areas. GP trainees are expected to become increasingly independent clinically over this year.

They are also expected, as part of their training, to take part in the local 'out-of-hours' arrangements. This might be based around the practice, a local cooperative (both of the former do still exist), or working with one of the commercial out-of-hours services. The RCGP is preparing to submit a case for extending training of general practitioners to the Department of Health.

Non-clinical skills for GPs – random rubbish or essential survival strategy?

One frequent complaint about ST3 'day release' teaching is that it can seem less focused on the MRCGP examination and more focused on things like communication and consultation skills, practice finances, the Quality and Outcomes Framework (QOF), leadership, involving the 'third sector' (voluntary organisations and charities), and ethics and professionalism. There will also usually be something on personality types and learning styles as well as some educational theory – general practice has become associated with medical education. There may also be a preoccupation with gatekeeping and commissioning skills. This section will briefly discuss gatekeeping, QOF and commissioning, to illustrate the relevance of thinking about these issues.

Gatekeeping

One of the key roles of any GP in the UK is as someone who can treat a range of conditions or refer patients on to specialist treatment. It is widely recognised that gatekeeping benefits both individual patients and the healthcare system. Individual patients benefit from having a personal doctor who can integrate their healthcare and view their problems together rather than in isolation. Patients as a whole benefit because the system ensures that expensive secondary care resources are spent on those who have the greatest need.

Some people, however, are concerned that gatekeeping can damage the doctor – patient relationship, since the doctor cannot act solely in the interests of the individual patient. Others have questioned whether this is ever possible, even without gatekeeping. Much depends on the system within which gatekeeping operates, and how great the pressures are on the primary care doctor *not* to refer, and how strong the incentives – personal, professional and financial – are for or against referral. There is a consensus that 'positive gatekeeping' in which doctors are rewarded for encouraging patients to have unnecessary or dubious procedures, as exists in many private systems, is unethical, and that avoiding unnecessary treatment is desirable.[5]

Two issues arising from the gatekeeping role of immediate importance to GPs are as follows:

- Does excessive referral by a GP to any particular specialty reflect a learning need in that area? If so, how will you address this? Does it reflect a problem or a particular demographic in a particular area (e.g. an elderly population)? Also remember that GPs receiving inducements for excessive referrals to any private service can now fall foul of the Bribery Act 2011 as well as the GMC!

- Under-referral is also hazardous. For example, GPs are perceived to be bad at spotting cancer early. Clinical negligence claims against general practitioners in the UK increased by nearly 20 per cent in 2010 compared with 2009, according to the Medical Defence Union (MDU), which indemnifies more than half of the GPs in the UK. The most common allegations were delayed or wrong diagnosis (60 per cent of notified claims) and failure to refer patients (15 por cent).

The Quality and Outcomes Framework

The QOF is an annual reward and incentive programme for all GP surgeries in England. The QOF contains four main components (caled domains): clinical, organisational, patient experience, and additional services. Each domain consists of a set of achievement measures, known as indicators, against which practices score points according to their level of achievement. The 2010/11 QOF measured achievement against 134 indicators; practices scored points on the basis of achievement against each indicator, up to a maximum of 1000 points.

- *Clinical care.* This domain consists of 86 indicators across 20 clinical areas (e.g. coronary heart disease, heart failure, hypertension) worth up to a maximum of 697 points.
- *Organisational.* This domain consists of 36 indicators (worth up to 167.5 points) across five organisational areas – records and information; information for patients; education and training; practice management and medicines management.
- *Patient experience.* This domain consists of three indicators (worth up to 91.5 points) that relate to length of consultations and to patient experience of access to GPs.
- *Additional services.* This domain consists of nine indicators across four service areas – cervical screening, child health surveillance, maternity service and contraceptive services.

The QOF gives an indication of the overall achievement of a surgery/ practice through a points system. Practices aim to deliver high-quality care across a range of areas for which they score points. Put simply, the higher the score, the higher the financial reward for the practice. The final payment is adjusted to take into account the surgery workload and the prevalence of chronic conditions in the practice's local area.

Issues you may want to consider:

- One of the ways in which practices avoid penalties is by reporting exceptions, such as patients refusing monitoring or medication.

- There are periodical alterations to which activities gain QOF points.
- Practices will often have at least one partner as a 'QOF lead' to monitor practice performance against targets. In real terms, practices with larger patient lists may find it harder to achieve targets.

Commissioning

This will be the hot topic for GPs depending on what changes take place in the NHS in 2012. Commissioning is more than just a resource allocation process, it involves four stages:

- identify the need (referred to as 'needs assessment')
- identify capacity to meet the need (referred to as 'tendering')
- deliver the service from that capacity (referred to as 'procurement')
- evaluate the service (referred to as 'contract management') – evaluation should be likened to ways of improving or replacing a service that is inadequate.

So GPs might want to consider how needs and priorities are identified, what process is involved in tendering and procuring, and how a service can be managed when it is not working. Perception of conflicts of interest means that providers of services in a locality should not have a role in directing commissioning groups.

Making the most of your ST3 year

The ST3 year is an opportunity to meet many different GPs in different practices on the vocational training schemes. Talk to your colleagues about their surgeries. If possible arrange a day or a week's exchange where you work in another practice which is sufficiently different from your placement. Get to know the practice you work in. This includes the non-clinical members of the team including the practice manager. Ask to sit in on practice and partners' meetings. This may involve staying late or missing a lunch but it will pay off.

Working hard and being committed is remembered, and a good reference from your training practice is essential. Find out what your ST3 practice needs as it may be able to link up your development needs with those of the practice you are in (Box 4.1). Many people choose their vocational training schemes in areas where they would consider settling down, and many practices have subsequently employed their registrar, whether as a locum, as a salaried GP or as a partner (since they like, know and trust them and have trained them).

- Minor surgery and joint injections
- Family planning
- Dermatology
- Child health
- Anticoagulation clinics
- Enhanced services (these attract extra payments for a practice, such as running a service for management of substance misuse)

Box 4.1 Key areas where you may gain valuable additional skills

From ST3 to qualification

Royal College of General Practice membership is now a compulsory exit qualification for all new GPs. It tests knowledge, skills and attitudes through workplace-based assessment, clinical skills assessment (an observed structured clinical examination), the applied knowledge test, and the requirement to submit a complete electronic portfolio of learning at the end of the training years.

GP trainees are assessed in the workplace and by examination: an applied knowledge test (AKT) and a clinical skills assessment (CSA). The AKT is a computer-marked timed examination aimed at assessment of relevant knowledge and reasoning – the knowledge is useful for the ST3 year so do not leave taking the exam until the last minute. The CSA is designed as a simulated GP surgery where role-players are used in the assessment of candidates' knowledge and consultation skills. The best practice for the CSA is seeing a lot of patients and doing a lot of consultation observation tools (see below). It is worth seeing the relevant training DVDs from the RCGP, and revision texts such as *Get Through MRCGP: Clinical Skills Assessment* may be of some use.

GP trainees are formally appraised by workplace-based assessment using two assessment tools: case-based discussion (CBD) (where a trainee presents a clinical case and discusses aspects of it with the educational supervisor) and the consultation observation tool (COT) (a formal method of assessing an observed consultation or video of a consultation between a trainee and patient). While it is no longer compulsory to use video in training and assessment, many trainees (and qualified GPs) find this useful in reflecting on their consultation skills. Trainees are guided to complete a minimum number of CBDs (and COTs). GP trainees in primary care undertake a case-based discussion with a trainer, who enters a record of the discussion, along with learning outcomes demonstrated and further learning goals into the trainee's e-portfolio. Critically the trainer may identify issues, which the trainee may have overlooked, or challenge a trainee's reasoning (Box 4.2).

- Don't be dismayed if at first trainers mark your efforts as inadequate. You will acquire knowledge and skills over the year.
- Use the e-portfolio to reflect on your clinical and non-clinical encounters so that you identify areas you need help with whilst an abundance of help is still available.

Box 4.2 Key tips with workplace-based assessments

The RCGP is reorganising the training curriculum for GPs to make it easier to navigate. The new curriculum, which launches in August 2012, comprises three parts: the core statement, called 'Being a GP'; the contextual statements; and the clinical examples.

Make use of online resources. e-GP (e-Learning for General Practice) is an online resource which provides GPs working in the NHS with a free programme of interactive e-learning modules. The resource was launched formally in July 2009. It contains a growing number of modules addressing a broad range of clinical and professional topics, based on the RCGP's curriculum for general practice. An automated link with the RCGP e-portfolio prompts the learner to record each completed session of learning and, by means of a reflective template, to reflect critically on the learning activity that has occurred and consider if this has revealed further learning priorities. Certified GPs may also use the tool as evidence for their annual appraisal.

GP-ST3s often grumble about having to fill in the e-portfolio. You need to get used to this, as it will make keeping up a portfolio for appraisal as a qualified GP much easier. At the end of the ST3 year you should have your first GP appraisal. This will count until the end of your first year as a new GP. Annual appraisal is a mandatory component of revalidation, which will start in 2012. Requirements for this include demonstrating that you have undergone 50 hours of CPD a year.

Life as a senior general practitioner

Partnership, salaried GPs, locums, urgent-care and out-of-hours GPs

Over the past 10 years the workforce in general practice has seen a noticeable shift: practices have begun taking on fewer general practitioner partners and instead are hiring more salaried GPs. Research conducted by the RCGP among its 'First Five' members – i.e. GPs in their first five years of practice after obtaining their certificate of completion of training (CCT) – found that only 23 per cent became partners within five years of qualifying, while 42 per cent were in salaried GP jobs and a quarter were working as locums.[6]

Under section 1 of the Partnership Act 1890, a partnership is defined as 'the relationship which subsists between persons carrying on a business in common with a view of profit'.

Not everyone seeks partnership. In many cases partners and salaried doctors do very similar roles clinically, but partners are required to take final responsibility when something goes wrong, and they carry the risk involved in running a general practice (Box 4.3). Partnership is a major commitment in terms of workload and finance, and when relationships break down between partners this can become very complicated. Some newly qualified GPs are keen to go straight into business as partners. Others prefer to spend a few years after qualification establishing their clinical and leadership skills and learning about the politics and business aspects of general practice before looking for a partnership.[7]

- More duties/responsibilities such as business and governance aspects of practice
- Extra meetings outside working hours
- QOF-related administration
- Dealing with practice-related problems
- Uncertain future of general practice: successive governments make changes to general practice
- Impact of extended hours and the possibility that GPs may go back to providing 24-hour cover for patients

Adapted from www.rcgp.org.uk

Box 4.3 Some drawbacks of partnerships

Salaried GPs can take on leadership roles in a practice or the local area. For example, a salaried GP might become involved with a practice's attainment of QOF targets or chair the practice's significant-event audit. Salaried GPs might take on a 'subspecialist role' such as running the practice's 6-week baby clinic, or diabetes review clinic. Salaried GPs and locums are also becoming involved in local commissioning of services and RCGP or BMA activities.

Locum work can be popular. After all, the rates of pay are often good, and the work can be arranged to suit the GP in terms of both time and geography. It is advisable to be as clear as possible in advance over what a practice expects from its locums. The BMA recommends agreeing this in writing.[8] Clarity involves avoiding surprises, such as finding out you are the sole GP in the practice or being handed a shopping basket-full of test results paperwork as you prepare to leave. At the very least establish whether you are expected to be the 'duty GP', or share duties such as visits or paperwork, as well as whether you are being paid an hourly or sessional rate. Be prepared to adjust your rates depending on the level of responsibility expected of you.

Since GP practices were able to relinquish out-of-hours cover in 2004 (usually from 6.30pm until 8.00am and weekends) two distinct types of general practice have emerged, which may employ new GPs on either a salaried or locum basis: 'urgent-care' and 'out-of-hours' general practices. Urgent Care Centre (UCC) GPs are often based in or linked to emergency departments and are employed to treat minor ailments or redirect non-acute problems back into main general practices (UCCs tend to see a lot of adult medicine and musculoskeletal medicine.) Out-of-hours (OOH) GPs essentially do what the GP 'on call' used to do. Visiting can involve a lot of care of the elderly, palliative medicine and mental health, whereas seeing patients at an OOH base can involve more acute paediatrics. An OOH telephone triage can involve allocating patients as a visiting or base appointment, reassurance, or calling an ambulance. There are many GPs who now work exclusively in the urgent-care or OOH setting.

Academic general practice

This is a valid career choice and not an oxymoron! Many academic GPs have split their time between research and practice. Some but not all also have involvement in undergraduate and postgraduate education (Box 4.4).

Links to academic departments can be found through the Society for Academic Primary Care, and further information on academic clinical fellowship programmes in general practice can be obtained from the National Institute for Health Research's Coordinating Centre for Research Capacity Development. Even if you are already a practising GP, it's not too late to consider an academic career.[9]

Most of the academic clinical fellowships, academic in-practice fellowships and clinical lectureship posts are research posts, although a minority are provided in medical education. Opportunities to get involved in general practice education exist in abundance (Box 4.5). All involve some form of training, and some may involve intensive training and separate appraisal. A number of institutions offer masters degrees and diplomas in medical education. The key organisations are the Association for the Study of Medical Education and the Academy of Medical Educators, which is formalising training and the career structure for medical education.

- Academic F2 placements in general practice: 4- month placements in foundation year 2
- Academic clinical fellowships for GP specialist trainees: extend current training to 4 years
- Academic in-practice fellowships for fully trained GPs: 2 years part-time masters-level training; Department of Health, Medical Research Council, Wellcome training fellowships; 3 years full-time equivalent, leading to a doctorate
- Clinical lectureships: for postdoctoral GPs, half time for up to 4 years
- Clinical senior lectureships: university, NHS, or joint funding, leading to a professorial post
- It is a pathway you can join or rejoin at various points, whether you are a student, trainee, or fully qualified GP

Adapted from http://careers.bmj.com/careers/advice/view-article.html?id=3008

Box 4.4 A career ladder for academic general practitioners

Financial considerations in general practice

There has been a perception that general practice has inferior clinical content but a superior lifestyle to hospital medicine.[10] Pay for GPs has fallen in real terms by 26.6 per cent since 2005/6. The real pay situation might be worse, as the figures show only the effects of inflation and pay awards on basic pay. Many other factors are currently having a detrimental effect on GPs' total remuneration, such as increasing costs of revalidation and the costs to general practices of registering with the Care Quality Commission (Box 4.6).[11] Moreover, changes to the indemnity cover of nurses in general practice (previously one of the roles of the Royal College of Nursing) may mean that practices have to pay for this as well.[12] If you are at all unsure about your entitlements in terms of expenses and tax it is highly advisable to engage an accountant, many of whom specialise in accounting for GP partners and locums.

Teaching medical students

- One-to-one as a GP tutor in your practice
- In groups as a seminar leader – there is a multitude of these including medical humanities, medical ethics, communications skills and clinical skills
- As an undergraduate course organiser for your local medical school

GP specialist trainees

- One-to-one as a GP trainer in your practice
- As a clinical supervisor out of hours
- As course organiser for your local training scheme
- As associate director or director of postgraduate GP education

Continuing medical education of GPs

- As a postgraduate centre GP tutor
- Both trainers and trainees groups will commission GPs with expertise in various areas to teach or facilitate a session on specialist topics

Adapted from http://careers.bmj.com/careers/advice/view-article.html?id=3008

Box 4.5 Educational roles for GPs

- Are drawings (share of profit paid to partners at regular intervals) fixed at monthly intervals?
- Does the practice's profit vary?
- Does the practice do cash-flow forecasting?
- Dispensing practices are higher earning.
- Teaching and training practices may earn less.
- There is a balance between number of patients and doing well on QOF.

Adapted from www.rcgp.org.uk

Box 4.6 Financial considerations in practice partnership

Applying for salaried GPs and partners positions

Questions you should ask

Are you choosing the right GP practice for you? Whether you are taking on a partnership or a salaried position you should ask yourself a number of questions:

- Do you know or like the area?
- Do you know or like the practice and the partners?
- Do you know or like the size of the practice?
- Are you looking for a teaching and training practice?
- Do you prefer a personal or shared list of patients?
- Does the practice include its partners and/or salaried clinicians in a group indemnity arrangement? Medical indemnity cover is a major tax-deductible expense for GPs.
- Is the practice profitable? This is more an issue if seeking partnership.
- Does the practice have a particular ethos? For example, some practices may have an overtly religious ethos, others may have a 'particular way of doing things'.
- How soon do new partners achieve parity? Parity is where new partners start on a lesser proportion of their share of practice profits, and gain a full share once they have taken a full share of partnership duties.
- If taking on a salaried position, do the duties include 'partnership' duties? If so, is there an understanding that partnership may be on offer at some point in the future?

Before applying for a partnership or a salaried position

- Find out about the practice. Does it achieve QOF targets?
- Arrange to visit the practice.
- Write a covering letter.
- Make sure you have a good, up-to-date CV and references.
- Consider telephoning the GP who is leaving, if shortlisted (asking about the pros and cons of working in the practice).
- Only apply for a partnership if you really want it and you think they may want you.

Establish what the practice wants

- How many sessions? Full time/part-time?
- Is there a commitment to teaching and/or training?
- What is the practice ethos?

You might consider asking the interviewers:

- What are the particular challenges of working in this practice?
- What can you offer this practice?

- What are the strengths of this practice?
- As with any job interview, always ask for feedback if you are unsuccessful.

Most GPs entering practice do so as an additional or replacement practitioner in an established partnership.[13] Prior to entering into any practice agreement as a partner, ask to see:

- an up-to-date partnership agreement
- a set of practice accounts.

You should be at liberty to seek independent legal or accountancy advice before committing to a partnership agreement. Be wary of joining a GP partnership that refuses access to the above or obstructs independent legal or accountancy advice.

New GP practices are still set up from scratch. Opportunities to do this may arise, for example, when towns expand, or when hospital trusts decide to have a GP surgery on site and open the project to tender. This is a rare but not an impossible undertaking that usually requires some expertise in both the initial bid and the project itself.

In summary

- Make the most of your ST3 year.
- There is no obligation to enter partnership immediately.
- Make the most of the MRCGP process.
- Make full use of the institutions you join. Both the RCGP and the BMA welcome motivated GPs who want to help shape the future of the profession.
- Be sure you apply for jobs that you want, and prepare beforehand.
- There is a variety of careers available within general practice.
- Good luck is enhanced by preparation!

References

1   Lorentzon M, Jarman B, Bajekal M (1994) *Report of the inner city task force of the Royal College of General Practitioners*. RCGP, London.

2   Deighan M (2008) Teaching about personal and professional responsibilities in the new curriculum. Chapter 16 in *General Practice Specialty Training: Making It Happen* (eds Mohanna K and Tavabie A), Royal College of General Practitioners, London.

3 Chana N (2008) Royal College of General Practitioners. Chapter 7 in *Choosing General Practice: Your Career Guide* (eds A Hastie and A Stephenson), BMJ – Blackwell, Oxford.

4 Papanikitas A (2011) Confidentiality and ethicality: an inverse care issue in general practice? *Clinical Ethics* **6(4)**: 186–90.

5 Toon P (2006) Ethics and family medicine. Chapter 8 in *European Textbook of Family Medicine* (eds NJ Mathers, G Maso and M Bisconcin), Passoni Editore, Milan.

6 Stirling A (2011) Less than a quarter of recently qualified GPs become partners in five years. *Pulse*, 23 May (www.pulsetoday.co.uk/newsarticle-content/-/article_display_list/12202627/less-than-a-quarter-of-recently-qualified-gps-become-partners-in-five-years).

7 Jaques H (2011) The GP partnerships debate. *BMJ Careers*, 6 December.

8 Jaques H (2011) Locums should agree terms in writing with employing practices. *BMJ Careers*, 2 November.

9 Kendrick T (2008) How about a career in academic general practice? *BMJ Careers*, 9 July.

10 Petchey R, Williams J, Baker M (1997) 'Ending up a GP': a qualitative study of junior doctors' perceptions of general practice as a career. *Family Practice*, 14(3): 194–8.

11 Jaques H (2011) Senior doctors' real-terms pay has eroded by up to 27 per cent in past six years. *BMJ Careers*, 26 November.

12 Jaques H (2011) GPs could bear cost of changes to nurse indemnity. *BMJ Careers*, 3 November.

13 Stanton T (2002) Choosing a practice. In *Succeeding in General Practice* (ed. I Bogle), pp. 27–41, Health Press, Abingdon.

Sources of further information

Academy of Medical Educators: www.medicaleducators.org

Association for the Study of Medical Education: www.asme.org.uk

British Medical Association GPC: More information about the General Practice Committee of the BMA can be obtained at: www.bma.org.uk/representation/branch_committees/general_prac/index.jsp

Good medical practice for GPs. A collaboration between the RCGP, the BMA GPC and the General Medical Council to identify specific standards and aspirations for general practice: www.rcgp.org.uk/pdf/PDS_Good_Medical_Practice_for_GPs_July_2008.pdf

InnovAIT: The RCGP journal that was developed to support Associates in Training (AiTs) of the RCGP from entry into specialist training to qualification. It is also a valuable resource for trained GPs who wish to update and maintain their knowledge base and newly qualified ('first five') GPs wanting to extend their knowledge: http://rcgp-innovait.oxfordjournals.org

National Association of Sessional GPs (NASGP): Supports freelance and locum GPs and its website is a useful source of practical advice for new GPs: www.nasgp.org.uk

National Institute for Health Research's Coordinating Centre for Research Capacity Development: www.nccrcd.nhs.uk

Quality and Outcomes Framework (QOF): www.qof.ic.nhs.uk

Royal College of General Practitioners: www.rcgp.org.uk/

Royal Society of Medicine GP and Primary Healthcare Section: A source of affordable update and CPD courses: www.rsm.ac.uk/gp

Society for Academic Primary Care: www.sapc.ac.uk

5

Managing your finances

Key aims of this chapter

- Give an overview of the areas of financial planning, including the NHS pension and its associated benefits, protection, mortgages, savings and the payment of tax
- Highlight the relevance of planning your finances and reviewing them on a regular basis, particularly as your career and life progress
- Outline the financial changes as you move from trainee towards senior doctor status.

Introduction

As you move through your training, life and your financial requirements will change. Income is likely to rise but so will expenditure. You may purchase a property or have a family, and with every change your financial needs arguably need to be reviewed. Even if you do not decide to 'settle down', you may find that a penchant for new cars and expensive holidays starts to increase at a higher rate than your salary! This chapter will cover each of the financial areas that may be relevant during your final (or ST) years of training through to your consultant or GP partner post and beyond.

Pensions

Pensions can appear very confusing, but some simple knowledge will clarify exactly where your contributions go and what to expect from them. It is important to note that many public sector pensions in the UK are currently under review. Almost all doctors contribute to the NHS pension which is available to all members of the NHS. You pay a percentage of your pensionable salary (does not include banding if applicable, but does include London weighting) as a monthly contribution in exchange for a pension at retirement, death benefits to your family or estate, and ill-health benefits in the event of incapacity ahead of your normal retirement age.

There are currently two parts to the NHS pension scheme: the 1995 section (Old Scheme) and the 2008 section (New Scheme).

The 1995 section

As a member of the pension scheme with service before April 2008 you are likely to be part of the 1995 section, which at present has a normal retirement age of 60 with a pension and lump sum. The standard lump sum is equal to three times the pension and currently is paid free of tax. You will accrue 1/80th of your final salary for every whole year you work, with the maximum being 45 calendar years of service. If you consider retirement before the age of 60 you will face an actuarial reduction to both the pension and lump sum (Table 5.1).

Lump sum

At retirement you currently have the option to commute income at a ratio of 1:12 to receive a larger lump sum, with the maximum being generally 5.36 times your pension including your standard lump sum. Note this would lead to a reduced income being paid for the remainder of your life, although any benefits payable to your dependants will continue to be based on the original higher pension.

Death benefits

In the event of an early demise, a death-in-service lump sum is payable equal to twice your final year's pensionable pay. The 1995 section will also provide an ongoing income to your spouse or civil partner for the remainder

Table 5.1: Actuarial reductions to pension and lump sum for retirement before the age of 60 under the 1995 section

Age	50	51	52	53	54	55	56	57	58	59
Pension (%)	60.2	62.9	65.9	69.0	72.5	76.3	80.4	84.8	89.6	94.7
Lump sum (%)	71.1	73.6	76.1	78.8	81.5	84.4	87.3	90.3	93.5	96.8

of their life. The survivor pension is paid at a rate equal to 50 per cent of an enhanced, or tier 2, ill-health pension (covered later in this chapter).

An allowance may also be payable to your dependent children if they are under the age of 23 and within full-time education or training and have been so continuously from the age of 17.

The 2008 section

Under NHS Pension Choice, every member of the 1995 section is given a one-off option to move into the new 2008 section. There are differences, and perhaps the most significant being the increase in the normal retirement age to 65 from 60. If benefits are taken from before the age of 65, an actuarial reduction will be applied (Table 5.2).

Note that within the 2008 section you accrue a pension but not a lump sum, although you may have a small amount of lump sum transferred across under the NHS Pension Choice exercise if you have moved from the 1995 section. At retirement you are able to commute income at the ratio of 1:12 to receive a lump sum, with the maximum generally 4.28 times your pension before the reduction to pay for the minimum lump sum. The benefits under the new scheme are enhanced to 1/60th for each year of service, compared with the 1/80th under the 1995 section.

The pension will be calculated using 'reckonable pay', which is the annual average of the best three consecutive years pay (pensionable) in the last ten years.

Death benefits

The 2008 section also provides benefits in the event of your early demise, although the calculations are different from those of the 1995 section. The death-in-service lump sum is twice your reckonable pay, and the survivor pension payable to your spouse or civil partner is 37.5 per cent (mathematically speaking, 50 per cent of the 1/80th pension is equal to 37.5 per cent of the 1/60th pension) of the pension you would have received had you retired through ill health on the day of your death.

Table 5.2: Actuarial reductions if benefits are taken before the age of 65 under the 2008 section

Age	55	56	57	58	59	60	61	62	63	64
Pension (%)	56.3	59.4	62.6	66.2	69.9	74.0	78.4	83.2	88.4	94.1

Membership records and accrued benefits

It is sensible to request an up-to-date Membership Statement on a regular basis, although the Pensions Agency will allow only one request in any 12-month period.

Checking the service details currently held by the Pensions Agency sooner and regularly will help to avoid service being 'lost' as Trusts change and records are erased. The easiest way to correlate your service is by comparing it with your CV with perhaps a second CV confirming the exact dates. An accrued benefit statement will also allow a degree of planning both in terms of expected pension and lump sum if applicable, along with the protection benefits that will continue to increase.

Income protection

Sick pay

Arguably the most important aspect of finance is your income. Unless you have very rich relatives or a partner who puts your medical salary to shame, then without your own salary everything would cease.

The NHS does provide sick-pay arrangements, and these gradually build to a maximum of 6 months' full pay followed by 6 months' half pay (Table 5.3). After that, potentially your income would fall to zero until returning to work in some capacity.

Retirement through ill health

If you are a member of the NHS pension scheme and have been a paying member for at least two years, and become permanently incapable of

Table 5.3: Sick pay entitlement (months) according to duration of service in the NHS

Service	Full pay	Half pay
<4 months	1	0
4 months–1 year	1	2
1–2 years	2	2
2–3 years	4	4
3–5 years	5	5
>5 years	6	6

doing your present job because of ill health, you may be able to receive a pension.

At present, ill-health retirement is split into two tiers:

- Tier 1 is entitlement to your accrued pension benefits without actuarial reduction for early payment. To qualify you must be accepted by the NHS medical advisers (currently Atos Healthcare in the UK) as being permanently incapable of doing your current NHS role.
- If you satisfy the requirements for Tier 2 entitlement, you will receive your accrued benefits to date enhanced by two-thirds of your prospective membership up to reaching your normal pension age. You will be deemed permanently incapable of both doing your current NHS role and permanently incapable of regular employment of like duration to your NHS post, taking account of your mental capacity, physical capacity, previous training and practical, professional and vocational training.

Index linking

If you are granted ill-health retirement, the benefits in payment will be increased year on year from April.

Returning to work with loss of pension

Although the definition for each tier of ill-health retirement requires the member to be permanently incapable of fulfilling his or her role, it is actually possible to return to work before normal retirement age – although limits are in place for both tiers, and in the case of Tier 2 retirement the enhancement may be lost.

If, after returning to work, you exceed the permitted level of total income including the pension payment, then your ill-health pension will be reduced and is known as 'abatement'.

Serious illness

In the devastating event that you are seriously ill and do not expect to live longer than 12 months, you can potentially apply to exchange all of your ill-health benefits for a one-off lump-sum payment. This will be calculated using exchange factors as follows:

1   Pension up to a level that gives the maximum permitted lump-sum amount (explained earlier) will be converted at the rate of £12 of lump sum for every £1 of pension given up.

2 The remaining pension will be converted to a lump sum at the rate of £5 for every £1 of pension.

Your dependants will still get any pension they are entitled to in full.

Permanent health insurance

What is it?

This income protection is an insurance policy that provides an income in the event of incapacity through illness or injury. Under current legislation, the benefits are paid tax-free as long as you have paid the monthly premiums.

There are a number of providers of permanent health insurance, so the next few paragraphs may help you to filter the options you consider most relevant. As a hospital doctor you are entitled to sick pay, with a maximum of 6 months' full pay followed by 6 months' half pay (see Table 5.3). If you are in receipt of your full pay in the event of incapacity, it is highly unlikely any insurer would provide any payment and would actually only start to make payments when your income halved, with a further 'top up' when your income ceased from the NHS.

It is therefore preferable to have waiting or deferred periods for any policy you consider that match the NHS sick-pay arrangements you have accrued to date. As you begin to generate private practice income, the cheques will often continue to arrive for several weeks after ceasing work due to illness. Thus, when considering covering any private income, give thought to how long income is likely to continue; the longer any deferred period is, the cheaper the monthly premium is likely to be.

Own- or suited-occupation definitions

This is arguably the most important decision when choosing an income protection provider. The easiest way to explain the difference is that, after years of training to work in your chosen specialty, falling ill could actually mean a claim is declined because you could fulfil *another role* in the case of a suited occupation.

On the other hand, if you are insured on an own-occupation basis and unable to perform your role due to illness or injury, then a claim is likely to be met. For example, for someone *insured as a general surgeon*, the loss of a digit could lead to being unable to operate and the definition would be met and a claim accepted.

Premiums – guaranteed or reviewable

At present within the marketplace you have the option to consider either 'guaranteed' or 'reviewable' premiums for your cover.

- If you opt for guaranteed premiums they will remain the same throughout the period of cover (although if your cover increases year on year then the premiums will increase to take this into account).
- If reviewable premiums are chosen, the insurer will have the option to increase (or decrease) your monthly premiums typically on a policy anniversary after the first 5 or 10 years.

If you have had an injury or illness since the inception of the policy and wish to consider moving providers (due perhaps to a premium increase), you are likely to find that the injury or illness will be taken into account by any new insurer and may lead to an increased premium or, worse still, an exclusion.

Cover to what age?

Insurance cover should ideally run to your normal retirement age; but, as already highlighted earlier in this chapter, that is likely to change with the revised NHS pension conditions.

If you suffer an illness or injury early in your career that leaves you unable to return to work, the policy will continue paying out until the end age or death.

As your career progresses and you continue to pay into the NHS pension scheme, you are building up pension benefits and potentially ill-health retirement benefits. If in the event of incapacity you receive an NHS ill-health retirement pension, it is very likely this will be taken into account by any insurance provider and the benefits potentially reduced.

It may well be that, towards the end of your career, the need for income protection is less – as your mortgage is cleared or significantly reduced, education costs have been covered, and your pension benefits have increased. At that point you may reconsider whether there is actually a need for the cover at all.

Private practice

Upon completion of your training, not only will your pensionable income increase, it is likely that in a number of specialties you will be able to work privately and generate further income.

It is also likely that your indemnity insurance costs will rise, particularly if you plan to work privately. You must inform your insurer of your intention to work privately. The level of income and your specialty will determine how much your annual premium will be.

You will have colleagues who work privately, some as individuals, others in groups or chambers. This will vary depending on where you are based. There are advantages to each. Working as an individual you will be able to choose exactly what you do and when you do it, whereas being part of a larger group could mean joint responsibility, the covering of holidays and sick days, and a share of the income – but also a degree of protection if you are the one away or too ill to work.

It is important to register with each of the private hospitals you intend to work at, along with each of the private medical insurers who will in most cases be settling your fees.

Finally, a good secretary can be invaluable, especially if you plan to work sizeable hours privately. As with NHS secretaries (and it could be the same person), yours will organise your diary, chase late payments of fees, assist with insurance documents for patients, and generally lessen the administrative burden.

Buying a property

The purchase of a property tends to be the highest expenditure most of us will make, whether it is your first flat or your perfect home upon becoming a consultant. The past few years have, to say the least, been interesting in the property market. There has been a trend away from 'gazumping', whereby a vendor might accept a higher offer at a late stage in the sale process, towards 'gazundering', whereby the purchaser offers a lower amount towards the date for exchange of contracts.

The deposit

The size of your available deposit for a property purchase is still the key. The greater the level of your deposit, the more choice of lenders and rates you will have. At the time of writing, 100 per cent mortgage loans were not available in the UK, although there is certainly an appetite from lenders to lend 90 per cent of the property's value.

There are many factors that will influence whether or not the deposit is sufficient, the first being your overall income and whether you are buying as an individual or as a couple.

All debts and liabilities will be taken into account by lenders, particularly loans and credit card balances, and these may reduce the amount available to borrow. If you are able to clear down debts in advance of purchasing a property, it is likely to leave a wider choice of lenders and potentially lower interest rate options – but do leave some savings for a deposit.

Mortgage types

If you are able to generate a sufficient deposit and find a property you want to purchase, it is then a question of what type of mortgage to seek. There are essentially two options: 'capital and interest' (repayment) or 'interest only'.

- *Repayment mortgage*. In brief, a repayment mortgage will see the outstanding capital (plus interest) reduced month on month throughout the term of the mortgage, until the balance is zero and the property becomes wholly yours. As long as you meet the monthly payments throughout the term, the mortgage will definitely be cleared.
- *Interest-only mortgage*. Here, you pay the mortgage lender only the interest portion of the loan each month and, at the end of the mortgage period, you are liable for the capital repayment *in full*. This final capital payment is usually met from the proceeds of the sale of the property, or some form of investment vehicle including the likes of ISAs, pension lump sums or life insurance. The danger is that the repayment of the loan is not guaranteed but is dependent on investment performance or prevailing property prices.

Choice of mortgage interest rate

A fixed rate

There are several options available when considering interest rates. The easiest to explain is the fixed rate. This will not vary during the fixed-rate term, which can be any period but typically is 2–5 years (although both shorter and longer fixed periods are often available). After the fixed rate expires the mortgage rate will become variable, until either a new fixed rate is agreed or until the end of the mortgage.

The tracker rate

This will literally track either the Bank of England's or the individual lender's base rate. As the rate being tracked varies, so will the interest rate you pay. For example, if you have a rate tracking the Bank of England's base rate (BBR) plus 2 per cent and the BBR is 0.5 per cent, you will pay an interest rate of 2.5 per cent; but if the BBR increases to 2 per cent then you will have to pay interest at 4 per cent.

The capped and collared rate

This is a variable type of interest rate that will increase or decrease as the BBR varies, but it has a ceiling point it cannot exceed as well as a floor it cannot fall below, regardless of whatever happens to the rate it is linked to.

Offset mortgages

To complicate matters further, there are offset mortgages. These actually allow you to 'offset' any savings you have against your outstanding mortgage balance. It will mean you can either reduce your monthly payments or shorten the term of your mortgage by keeping payments at the same level without funds offset. For example, if you had a mortgage of £200 000 with savings of £10 000 offset, you would only need to pay the monthly payment assuming a £190 000 debt; or you could keep the payment the same as if you had £200 000 outstanding, for a shorter period.

The mortgage application process

Finding the right property is often the most difficult part (although by the end of the process it may not seem it). You then have to agree a purchase price. If an offer you make is declined it may be appropriate to increase your offer (assuming you still want the property), but in ever decreasing increments – for example, a declined offer of £200 000, then £210 000, then £215 000, until the vendor accepts or declines the highest offer you are prepared to make.

You then need to decide what type of mortgage and interest rate you prefer and submit an application to the chosen lender. The mortgage lender will then financially underwrite you, taking into account your credit history, income and any debts or liabilities. The lender will typically require copies of your payslips, bank statements and, in some cases, proof of a deposit capability.

An independent valuation of the property will be required by the lender, although in almost every case you will pay for this valuation. This necessitates a survey of the property, of which there are three types:

- *Mortgage valuation survey.* Usually the surveyor will use comparisons from local house sales to provide an estimated value to the property. Normally this will contain a description of the house, confirmation of whether any special reports are required, as well as a general description of the condition of the property. This can include issues such as structural movement or damp walls or floors.
- *Homebuyer report.* The report is written in a standard format and is around 25 pages in length. It is more comprehensive than the standard valuation and focuses on essentials (e.g. urgent or significant defects and problems that may affect the value of the property). The report is typically more expensive than a mortgage valuation but less expensive than a structural survey.
- *Structural survey.* This is suitable for all residential properties and provides a full picture of the construction and condition, including the roofs, chimneys, walls, floors, ceilings, doors and windows (and an asbestos check). It is more likely to be needed if the property is, for example, of unusual construction, dilapidated or altered, or where a major renovation or conversion is planned.

Legal aspects of the purchase

You will choose a firm of solicitors to act on your behalf for the purchase. Check they are acceptable to the lender from the outset, to avoid the payment of unnecessary fees.

Your solicitor will carry out registry checks to confirm, for example, that the property is the vendor's to sell, and that a new motorway is not planned through the garden!

Once the mortgage and valuation checks are complete, a 'mortgage offer' will be sent out. This should confirm all details of the mortgage and property value, including the interest rate, monthly payments and the term of the mortgage. You will need to return a signed copy of the mortgage offer, and your solicitor will oversee an exchange of contracts. This is the point at which you typically transfer some or all of the deposit along with confirmation that you are buying the property and that the vendor is selling. The next step is completion, when the mortgage fund is transferred from your solicitor to the vendor's solicitor, and you receive a set of keys in exchange!

Family protection

Individuals view the need for financial protection very differently. Some insure just about everything – themselves, their pets, the house, car, phone, anything and everything. Others prefer to insure the essentials only (which in the case of owning a property would be the building) and the car for those who drive it. The ideal probably lies somewhere in between and will change throughout your career.

As an FY1, the need for life cover, income protection or critical illness cover isn't something the majority rush to consider, although ironically everything tends to be cheaper because of younger age and relative lack of a medical history. As you move through from FY to ST, your needs will certainly begin to change, particularly if you start a family. Combine that with the purchase of a property and you have moved from being seemingly carefree to having significant responsibilities. As mentioned earlier, the NHS will provide some cover, but it is unlikely to be sufficient particularly early in your career.

Life insurance

Life cover will provide a lump sum, ongoing income, or both, in the event of your death.

Spouse/partner survival

If you are financially interlinked with a spouse or partner then you should consider how things would function financially in the event of the death of one of you. If one income is significantly higher than the other the impact could be severe. The provision of a lump sum to provide an ongoing income for life, combined with any NHS benefits payable, can allow the continuation of a lifestyle.

Mortgage liability

If you have a mortgage or significant other liabilities, your life cover should provide the survivor (or your estate) with the ability to clear the debt and therefore lessen the ongoing burden for those left behind. Cover associated with a mortgage should ideally mirror the outstanding debt, term and type of mortgage (repayment or interest-only).

Dependants

If you have a family, the provision of an ongoing income specifically for the children could be used to cover the likes of childcare during the earlier years and education costs later on. This type of plan would normally have a specific term from the outset, ideally to the end of the children's education.

Critical illness cover

Critical illness policies can provide cover literally for the whole of your life or just for a set term, such as while you still have a mortgage. However, in contrast to life cover where it is relatively easy to organise a claim upon proof of death, critical illness cover is a little more complex.

There are a number of providers of this type of insurance offering both reviewable and guaranteed premiums with numerous conditions covered. Life cover can be included on the same plan; so, in the event of an individual suffering any one of the illnesses covered within the plan definitions, a payout would be made even if death did not occur.

Always check the policy details and make sure the plan covers the areas you are concerned about.

Debts and savings

Coping with debts

During the early years of most careers in medicine the majority of doctors tend to have negative savings, sadly as a result of student loans, a graduate loan and the use of credit cards. Painful as it may be, writing down the debts you have – including the amounts outstanding, the monthly payments and interest rates – will allow you to prioritise repayment of the debts with the highest interest rates first. The sooner you pay down a debt the less interest you will actually pay. However, check whether any penalties or early repayment charges apply in the event of the debt being settled ahead of the original end date.

Managing your savings

If you are fortunate enough to have some savings, it is important that you try to maintain a contingency fund to allow for financial emergencies. Ideally the funds should be available immediately. A sum equal to approximately three times your monthly expenditure should be held, although this will be very much a personal choice. Some prefer considerably more and others rely on credit cards – which can lead to further interest and debt issues.

If funds are kept within an interest-paying account, you will be liable to pay tax on interest received. If you do have savings, a tax-efficient way of holding them is within ISAs, which are in two forms: cash, and stocks and shares. The combined limit for the tax year 2011/12 is £10680, although a maximum of £5340 only can be within a cash ISA. If you consider investing in ISAs, outline your timeline and ensure you review your attitude to risk, understanding the potential downsides, be it inflation exceeding the returns or the value of your investments actually falling.

If your savings are to be used to fund a deposit for a property purchase, it would be wise to consider less adventurous options. Cash ISAs should ensure the funds do not decrease in value (although if held for significant time, inflation will potentially erode the 'real' value). The interest rates available vary from provider to provider, so be sure to check the returns available along with any restrictions on withdrawing your funds, and when the interest is actually added to your account. An annual payment may not suit if you plan to use the savings within a year.

The Financial Services Compensation Scheme

Your savings are protected under this scheme. The level of protection for deposit-type accounts is currently £85000 per person *per organisation*. If you have multiple accounts with various companies, be sure to check that they are not part of the same authorised institution.

Taxation

As an employee of a Trust you will pay tax on a pay-as-you-earn (PAYE) basis, so the amount you receive in your account each month should be after all the necessary deductions. However, it is wise to check your payslip and the tax code you currently have. A typical tax code is three numbers followed by the letter L, such as 747L. This would suggest you can earn up to £7475 of income before being liable for tax – known as your 'personal allowance'.

If your tax code ends with a different letter it could be that you have previously underpaid tax, or perhaps you could be overpaying now. It is likely to be a simple error between payroll departments with regard to your total income for a tax year, so it is important you keep any P45 or P60 you receive from employers and forward them to the payroll department at the new Trust upon arrival.

Record keeping

Depending upon your chosen specialty, you may receive crematorium fees or work locum sessions, and you may also generate income from account interest or the renting out of a property. Whatever income you generate, keep a record as it will be required when you file a tax return.

Also keep a record of expenses incurred in connection with your roles, be it GMC registration, parking for a locum session or membership of the various colleges and journals. Essential expenses will lessen the overall income level you are liable to pay tax on.

The tax return

It is likely that you will remain a higher rate taxpayer throughout your working life and into retirement, so you should consider filing a tax return every year.

You can file a tax return yourself, either online or using a paper form (the deadlines differ). Alternatively you may wish to engage an accountant to complete the documentation for you and assist with any difficulties. There will be fees involved, but the accountant should lessen the stress of filing a tax return. Moreover, if you employ a specialist medical accountant, he or she will look to submit relevant expenses, including journals subscriptions, college memberships, etc. Proper business expenses could see the actual revenue reduced by 40 or even 50 per cent, depending on your tax rate.

As you move into a consultant or senior GP post, particularly if you generate private practice income, a specialist accountant can be invaluable. He or she can advise on the most efficient ways of drawing income and offsetting potential expenses.

Sources of further information

BMA pensions advice: www.bma.org.uk/employmentandcontracts/pensions

Financial Services Compensation Scheme: www.fscs.org.uk

HM Income Tax office: www.hmrc.gov.uk/incometax/index.htm

HM Revenue & Customs: www.hmrc.gov.uk

6

Conferences, courses and networking skills

Key aims of this chapter

- Give an overview of conference types available to clinicians
- Discuss study leave and attendance at courses
- Explore ways to develop networking skills.

Introduction

During specialist training there will be ample time to attend courses and conferences both in the UK and abroad. This represents an opportunity to display posters or give presentations and you should do this if you can. This might be of data from a GP audit, information on new hospital guidelines, a case series, or data from a research project.

Attending conferences can be costly and, with study leave budgets being cut, you need to choose and plan wisely which conferences you attend. You might also need to use some of your study budget and leave to attend courses for both postgraduate exams and specialist courses to further your career, such as a management or teaching course.

As you become a more senior doctor and attend conferences more frequently, it is vital that you keep in touch with people you have met along the way. Building up professional relationships is important, as you never know when a contact could be useful. After all, the next time you meet that consultant you had a drink with at the conference bar may just be when he or she sits opposite you on an interview panel!

Attending conferences

Study leave

The NHS is currently undergoing intensive financial scrutiny, and this situation is unlikely to improve in the near future. A number of hospital Trusts are cutting back on study leave funding, so it is important that you find out exactly how much money and how much leave you are entitled to in any new post. Hospitals have to provide a study leave budget for all doctors in training positions. This does not apply to doctors in non-training posts or Foundation Year 1 doctors. This leave needs to be approved by your consultant or department head a significant time in advance (e.g. 6 weeks), before being sent on to be approved by the relevant managerial department.

Additionally, you need to show evidence on the application form that the course is to further your own education. This may be in terms of a postgraduate course to prepare for exams or a specialist training course. Some Trusts will ask for additional information – such as confirmation that you have read a relevant paper before attending a specialist revision course, or that you have been revising for a specific exam before going on a course.

Funding will vary depending on your level of seniority, but as a rough guide you can expect somewhere between £400 and £800 a year to spend on courses. This figure can also be used for travel or accommodation where appropriate. Often, though, there will be strict policies to adhere to (e.g. that funds cannot be spent on conference dinners or alcohol). The length of study leave also varies between 10 days to 4 weeks a year, in addition to any in-house study leave that is mandatory for doctors in training – such as advanced life support courses and specialist training days.

Finally, if there is a course that you particularly want to go on, the onus will be on you to swap out of any on-calls and make sure your other commitments, such as clinics and operating lists, are adequately covered. You will have to stipulate on the leave form that you have organised all this.

Types of conference

Clinical conferences occur in every specialty. By the time you have reached ST level you should be familiar with some of them and may even have attended a few. There will often be UK, European and US versions of the same conference. For example, a UK chest doctor could attend the British Thoracic Society meeting, European Respiratory Society meeting or American Thoracic Society meeting. In addition to these general specialty-specific conferences, there will be a number of more specialised conferences, often with strange names; for example, the 'acid-fast club' meet twice a year to discuss tuberculosis research.

Clinical conferences also have a large social aspect to them. The main ones within a specialty are often frequented by the same people, and senior clinicians use this as an opportunity to meet and catch up with the gossip. It can be an important place to talk about jobs, fellowships and other training opportunities. However, be warned as there is little more damaging to your future career than dancing on tables at the conference bar in front of your prospective consultant colleagues. Other social events will be organised by sponsors of the conference, such as drug companies or those selling medical equipment. These can be signed up for in advance, so try to find out where and when they are happening.

Funding streams

In addition to funding, it is possible to get sponsorship from a number of other avenues to cover the conference registration fees, travel and accommodation. To be eligible, you may have to show evidence of having submitted an abstract or have been selected to present your data in the form of a poster or oral presentation. Conference organisers may have details of their own travel awards for individuals, especially for more junior and first-time attendees. These will be detailed on their website. They will also have links to the conference sponsors themselves who may have funding earmarked to invite doctors to attend the conference 'on their behalf'. Your deanery will have additional travel money available for some trainees to attend the major conferences. Finally, it is worth scoping out potential charities and other organisations that may have funding. For example, the British Lung Foundation and Asthma UK both currently give travel awards to doctors who wish to travel to the European Respiratory Society or American Thoracic Society meetings.

There are other types of conference that you may wish to attend, such as scientific conferences, and you can use your study leave and budget towards these. These types of conference may be useful to you particularly if you are thinking of studying for a higher research degree, so it is appropriate to attend a scientific meeting in your area of interest to help you with research applications. Alternatively, it may be that you have finished your time in research but want to still keep a hand in, or that you want to attend to present your research data. If you are interested in management you should consider attending a conference suited to doctors wishing to study current NHS policy. You may be interested in medical education and find there are many opportunities both in the UK and abroad to attend meetings, such as the annual meeting of the Association for the Study of Medical Education (ASME).

Conference fees

Clinical and scientific conferences have a variety of attendance fees. For example, students and junior doctors may pay less than senior doctors. There may also be a discount if you have been selected to present your work (see below), or if you are going to a meeting held by an organisation of which you are already a fee-paying member. Finally, there may be different prices depending on when you register: an 'early bird' price (the cheapest) which may be months in advance of the meeting, a regular price, and then a more expensive price as the conference date approaches. This is often difficult to decide, and potentially therefore more expensive, for trainees who do not know their rota months in advance.

Posters and presentations

To have the best chance of securing funding to attend a conference, and to boost your CV, it is worth submitting an abstract to the meeting you wish to attend. Abstracts can be submitted for most clinical and scientific conferences, and details of exactly how to do this will be on the conference website. Often they will be short (200–300 words), similar in length to the abstract of a paper. For large conferences, the majority of submitted abstracts will be chosen as it gives the meeting organisers a chance to boost their attendance numbers. In fact, you often have to specify on the submission form that you are definitely going to attend (or that you have already registered for the meeting) once your abstract is selected.

The date for decision making about whether or not your abstract is selected will be given in advance of the final date of registration, thereby allowing you to decide whether or not to attend the meeting. When submitting, you may be asked to decide whether to submit your abstract as a poster or a talk. In some cases, the conference organisers will make this decision for you.

Posters will be on display at various sessions throughout the conference. These may be during lunch or coffee breaks. However, for the larger conferences, there will be dedicated poster sessions. The posters will have to be a certain size, may have to be either landscape or portrait only, and there may even be rules about the font size and background colours. If you have been selected to give a talk, this will usually be for a short period, with similar talks grouped together (e.g. an afternoon of congenital heart defect talks during a cardiology conference). As with the posters, there will be rules to adhere to, such as time limits that will be enforced by a chair person.

If you feel that your work deserves more exposure than a poster or a brief talk, you may be able to give a longer presentation. These are usually given by the more senior members in the field and most will be invited talks; but keep an eye out on the website where the organisers may have an open invite asking for potential speakers to discuss their data. Finally, most conferences have late-breaking abstract entries. These are reserved for more important pieces of communication and can be submitted close to the meeting date. They may also be associated with prizes or travel funding, so it is worth keeping an eye out for these.

Courses to further your career

Exam preparation courses

These courses are very popular among trainees sitting postgraduate exams, but it is important to choose them wisely as they can be expensive. They have the potential to make a lot of money for the course organisers, so they are often marketed very heavily with advertising in a number of journals and hospital magazines. Before parting with your hard-earned cash it is worth speaking to people who have sat the exams before you and attended the courses. The best courses are often full simply because of their reputation and you should try and attend these as a priority.

Courses for written parts of postgraduate exams may simply focus on MCQs or short-answer questions as appropriate. They are often held in large lecture halls to get as many candidates in as possible. You will usually be given written material and course handouts, and these may be available prior to starting the course to allow you some background reading. You may also be given access to online exam materials including banks of past questions. In addition, these online areas may be charged extra to the course, so it is important that you find this out before booking.

Practical parts of postgraduate exams have their own specific courses and these can be extremely expensive. The main reason for this is that, unlike courses to prepare for the written exam, practical courses will need to pay for patients and other volunteers (e.g. actors to come and be examined by candidates), as well as multiple examiners. Courses involving practical techniques also need the equipment as well as the expertise to teach them. As with courses for the written exam, the best courses will book out early, so plan well in advance. Many candidates go on multiple courses at considerable personal expense, and in the long run this could be the cheaper option (both financially and emotionally) when compared to having to re-sit the exam. Importantly, however, going on a course is not imperative for success in the exam and you should not feel pressurised to go on one.

Interview preparation courses

These are discussed in detail in Chapter 13. They can be valuable in terms of improving your confidence when faced with an important interview. However, in a real interview you should be wary of giving repetitive answers that sound as though they have been learned by rote. Potential interviewers will want to see a line of thinking in order to get to an answer or an opinion, rather than simply reading back a pre-thought-out statement.

Practical procedure courses

These can be very useful for doctors who have been out of practice for a while (e.g. in research or on maternity leave), for those wishing to learn new and advanced techniques, or for those who simply want to brush up their existing knowledge. These courses are advertised widely but they can be expensive, depending on their exact nature, and so it is worth reading reviews and speaking to people who have been on such a course. They may use real patients (e.g. if learning to ultrasound pleural effusions) or models (e.g. for central line placement under ultrasound guidance). In reality, there is no substitute for simply doing the procedure yourself (under supervision) in a real clinical setting. However, some procedure courses can be helpful as an adjunct to this.

Specialist courses

In addition to the routine courses that all doctors will do in their training, there will be a number of specialist courses available. In all cases, you should decide what type of senior doctor you wish to be before pursuing such courses in your spare time. For example, if you want to be an academic clinician with a grounding in genetics then it is worth pursuing advanced scientific training in this area. On the other hand, if you are a GP with an interest in management, you may wish to pursue courses related to the NHS Confederation (see the end of this chapter for a link).

Finally, remember that your free time is limited, so always ask yourself two questions when applying for any course:

- Is it worth your money?
- Is it worth your time?

If the answer to either of these questions is no, then you may be better off doing something else in your free time.

Networking

What is networking?

Networking is simply an umbrella term for meeting people and getting to know them a little better, in either a professional or a social setting. The aim is often to further develop your professional career simply by making contacts that you can then follow up in the long term. These people may put you in touch with others who can help you, they may need help themselves, or they may simply become colleagues to whom you can go for advice.

Social networking (Facebook, Twitter, doctors.net.uk etc.) is simply a modern method of developing and keeping contacts. However, as outlined by the British Medical Association's guidance (see the end of this chapter for a link), they can contain a number of useful pieces of information. The key points from the current BMA guidance are given in Box 6.1.

Fifteen tips for successful networking

Be curious

When meeting someone for the first time, one of the best ways to start is by asking a little about themself. For example, if you find yourself at a small group discussion in a conference you may want to start up a conversation with your fellow medics. Ask them what they do and where they are from. Appear genuinely interested and they may be willing to talk to you. This is a far better method than starting conversations by simply talking about yourself.

Discuss mutual experiences and common ground

Medicine is a very small world. If you are at a national conference within your own specialty it is likely that you have mutual acquaintances, have

- Social media can blur the boundary between an individual's public and professional lives.
- Doctors and medical students should consider adopting conservative privacy settings where these are available, but be aware that not all information can be protected on the web.
- The ethical and legal duty to protect patient confidentiality applies equally on the internet as to other media.
- It would be inappropriate to post informal, personal or derogatory comments about patients or colleagues on public internet forums.
- Doctors and medical students who post online have an ethical obligation to declare any conflicts of interest.
- The BMA recommends that doctors and medical students should not accept Facebook friend requests from current or former patients.
- Defamation law can apply to any comments posted on the web made in either a personal or professional capacity.
- Doctors and medical students should be conscious of their online image and how it may impact on their professional standing.

Box 6.1 Key points from the BMA guidance on social networking

similar backgrounds or may have even worked with the same people. Try and explore these, as it will allow you to get to know a person better in the early stages.

Have the elevator pitch ready

This is a brief but important summary of your life (i.e. one you could give in the limited time of a moving elevator) and ambitions and can be changed as needed. For example, if you are a surgical trainee with a research background your brief pitch may have a similar theme but the content may be very different when speaking to a research professor compared with a full-time NHS consultant. You should know when to use either pitch and have it ready when asked.

Offer them something in return

Rather than simply trying to find out what you can gain from a situation, try to see if they need anything. For example, if you are chatting to a consultant who is looking to offer a new consultant job, then offer to spread the word to people who may be interested in applying. This means that they are more likely to remember you in the future.

Make a note of the person and their position

If you meet someone new who you think could be worth knowing for the future, make a note of his or her position and contact details. Few doctors use business cards (other than when trying to drum up private practice), but work emails should be readily accessible through the internet (e.g. by simply searching on a hospital Trust website) provided they are happy for you to contact them. There are a number of web databases and phone apps to allow you to keep a 'rolodex' of contacts, and it is important that you keep this up to date.

Remember quirks about people you meet

It is worth trying to make a note of other facts about people you meet. If they mention that they are moving to a new job, talk about their children or discuss a recent holiday that they enjoyed, then try to make a note of this too. Little details like this can prove invaluable when you meet again in the future, as they will think that you have genuinely paid attention to them when you first met.

Do not appear eager for a job

Don't be pushy for a job, even if that may be your main goal for forging a professional relationship. It is far better to appear cool about job prospects but at the same time remain interested in any upcoming positions. If there is a particular job or position you are interested in, then by all means let the person involved know of your interest – but don't push too hard as it will only turn people off.

Don't sell yourself too much but don't undersell yourself either

This is a difficult tip but some doctors are very good at it. When asked about yourself you should try to be keen and talk about your skills, experience and attributes. However, there is a fine line between appearing keen and being pushy. Doctors are naturally wary of salespeople, so if you find that you are starting to sound as though you are selling a used car then dial back the enthusiasm.

Ask them if they have anyone else in the field you can speak to

The majority of doctors you meet at conferences, courses or in social settings will have contacts that may be of use to you in your future career. For example, if you are interested in interventional endoscopy then it is worth asking gastroenterologists who they would recommend you speak to and ask more questions about the technique and how you could get trained in it. Even if they don't have any contacts themselves, they may be able to point you in the direction of someone who does.

Contact people who you are referred to as soon as possible

If you are introduced to new contacts, then try to speak to them sooner rather than later. This is important as you then have a recent timeframe within which to find some common ground; for example: 'I met your registrar at last month's conference and she suggested I talk to you about fellowships in your department.'

Don't commit to something that you cannot follow through

This is an important tip as nobody likes a timewaster. Don't say that you can help someone with a problem and then not follow through. This will simply give you a bad reputation and mean that people won't offer to help you in the future. It is far better to tell someone upfront that you cannot help them rather than to promise something that you cannot deliver.

Form alliances

Networking can be a lonely process, especially if you are hunting for a job or particular position such as a fellowship or research opportunity. It may be of some advantage to team up with colleagues. Try to share contacts and you will find that, between a group of trainees, you will have a number of avenues to further your own career.

Be smart

This applies to your dress code rather than anything else. At conferences and other meetings be as smart as possible. You might not want to wear a suit when perusing posters in the lunch session, but smart trousers and a shirt make a much better impression when you meet new people than wearing jeans and a T-shirt. Unfortunately, people may remember you more for your appearance than your experience, so save the Hawaiian shirts for when you make professor.

Think quality, not quantity

As important as it is to have many contacts, in medicine it is often better to have fewer but better ones than a large number of less helpful contacts. In crude terms, it may be better to be on first-name terms with one professor in your deanery than with two hospital consultants.

Build long-term relationships

The most important thing about building up professional contacts is that you make lasting relationships. By continuously meeting people in your training region and trying to maintain contact with them, you will be able to develop contacts that can help you at every stage in your career. Like plants, your relationships need to be gently tended from time to time but otherwise be left to grow by themselves until a time when you really need their help.

Sources of further information

BMA social media guidance: www.bma.org.uk/images/socialmediaguidancemay2011_tcm41-206859.pdf

Networking from NHS Connecting For Health: www.connectingforhealth.nhs.uk/systemsandservices/icd/informspec/careerplan/phi/personal/learningweb/personal/networking

NHS Confederation: www.nhsconfed.org/Pages/home.aspx

7

Research: getting in

Key aims of this chapter

- Give an overview of the reasons for undertaking research
- Explain the funding opportunities available to clinicians
- Explore the fundamentals of clinical academic research.

Introduction

A number of readers will have been exposed to research as an undergraduate. This might have been part of a bachelor of sciences degree or simply as a project during a basic sciences degree, clinical attachment or specialty module. This exposure sometimes puts clinicians off research for life, but for a few the appeal of research may be more long term.

For those who have not been previously exposed to research, it can be very difficult to get into and can also be very confusing. Should you apply for a grant from the Medical Research Council, or should you apply directly to a research group? Should you take up the post for one year, or should you apply for a three-year PhD? Should you work in the clinical side of research (e.g. investigating a new asthma inhaler), or do you have the skills to tackle the subject from a basic science point of view? These are interesting questions because different types of research are suited to different types of people.

In the current jobs climate it is important to consider doing research either to pursue an academic career or simply to stand out from your colleagues and for progression along your chosen career pathway. In this chapter we discuss the merits of different types of research as well as the best way to approach getting into research.

Finding out about research opportunities

Finding a suitable supervisor

The best way to decide what type of research to undertake is to meet people and talk about the opportunities available to you. All clinical institutions have some level of research, and the bigger teaching hospitals which are closely affiliated with universities have active scientific collaborations. The first place to start will be at the universities.

Getting involved can be as easy as finding an area that interests you and phoning the relevant departmental head. Most academic researchers are very approachable and keen to support young inquisitive minds, especially if you are interested in their area of work.

Prior to meeting any potential supervisor, you should read up about the academic area of interest and the research interests of their group. Review the university's website where there will be a brief biosketch listing their main achievements and future goals in their particular area of research. There will also be a list of funding streams supporting their research, as well as a record of their publications. Try to familiarise yourself with their most important and their most recent papers, even if it means simply reading the abstracts. Also read a little around their field of work to see what their main competitors are up to, and try and identify ways in which you could fit into their group.

Once you have arranged a meeting through the group's secretary or personal assistant, make sure you dress smartly (as if for an interview) and arrive on time. Be prepared to have a working meeting as most academics are very busy. Even if they can spend half an hour with you to discuss research opportunities, they may make phone calls, send emails or even discuss issues with their group at the same time. Make sure you have sent them an electronic copy of your CV, but take along a paper copy as often they won't have time to read it or print it out.

Use this time wisely. For example, make sure you ask the right questions, appear enthusiastic and try and show that you have some understanding of the work going on within the research group. Ask about the future directions of the group to show that you have thought about working with them.

In reality, it is very unlikely that research funding will be available to make it possible for you to join the group immediately. However, professors and other academics are always on the lookout for new funding opportunities, so if you appear enthusiastic and intelligent they may make a note to write your potential salary into an upcoming grant proposal. Alternatively, they may contact colleagues in related fields on your behalf to see where funding is available and put you in the right direction. The most important thing is to be enthusiastic – academics are always keen to encourage an interest in academic medicine amongst younger doctors.

Choosing a supervisor

If you are fortunate enough to obtain funding to do research, it is vital that you choose both the group and the supervisor carefully. Young and dynamic professors may be very exciting to work for and may also be able to give you a lot more time in terms of supervision than the more established, famous professors. However, it may be that the more established professors are better at getting funding and consequently have more equipment and staff to help you with your own work.

It is also important to make the distinction between a clinical academic and a basic scientist. Clinicians may be more useful in terms of long-term contacts and networking within your own speciality. However, a basic scientist may, in some cases, have a better grasp of the fundamentals of that particular subject. When starting your research degree it is vital that you learn and develop these basics skills from the very beginning and have an important grasp of the fundamentals of research, such as research ethics, before trying to tackle the bigger picture.

You may need to meet with a number of academics – for example the first scientist you meet may not be the right one to guide you through your own research – and you may have to meet a number of other people before finding the right environment for you.

The group that you choose is also important. A small intimate group with a few scientists may be a very warm and nurturing environment to work in, and one that is supportive so that you get the right guidance throughout your research time. A larger group may have more equipment and facilities, but may be more impersonal – and you might find that people are competing for equipment time, which can be quite daunting at first.

Finally, remember that good research occurs both within and outside the UK. A number of the most important diseases affecting the global population – such as HIV infection, malaria and tuberculosis – may be best studied in parts of the world where they are endemic. This type of research is often looked upon favourably by grant bodies, particularly if it occurs under the supervision of an academic based in the UK.

Types of research

There are a number of different types of research, and it is vital that if you are going to spend one to three years of your life in a single area that you choose the correct one.

In simple terms, research can currently be divided up into three broad areas: basic science, translational research and clinical research.

- Basic science research involves tackling a specific hypothesis using a wide range of laboratory techniques, even though the work itself may be on clinical samples. This may involve animal work, so it is important that you understand the ethical implications of this as well as explore your own perceptions towards animal experimentation before you embark on such research.
- Translational research involves translating basic science principles into the clinical setting (or vice versa). However, it can be very difficult to jump into translational work at a junior level, so it may be better to commit yourself to another type of research to start with. For example, a junior clinical academic may spend five years investigating a novel asthma pathway and then become a lead researcher and spend the next ten years trying to develop a novel drug based on this pathway.
- Clinical research can be exciting and is often considered more rewarding as it can have a more real immediate impact. It can be as diverse as investigating a new device in a surgical setting to reviewing large amounts of epidemiological data to create mathematical models.

Once you have chosen the type of research you want to do, you need to choose a specific area to research in. For example, if you are a cardiologist and you want to perform research, you could choose one of the biggest topics in cardiology, such as heart failure or angina. These will have the most funding available, but they will also potentially be the most competitive to get into because a lot of people may be doing very good research in these areas. You may therefore wish to choose a slightly more esoteric condition, such as cardiac amyloidosis. This may be harder to fund in the long term than research into heart failure, but it might mean that if you do pursue an academic career then you could become one of the few specialists nationally and internationally in this field. Whatever type and area of research you decide upon, it is vital that you choose wisely as you may spend the rest of your life working on that particular topic.

Research degrees

Research can be performed part-time or full time and can range from simple one-week attachments in an area to a research degree, such as an MD or PhD. Short attachments or periods in research are useful if you have no research training or background, as this will allow you to become familiar with a research group and enable you to meet people with a number of different skills. It may also be enough to show you that you do not want to pursue a research career after all.

Research can also take the form of small projects or fellowships, and the latter is discussed further in Chapter 11.

In terms of formal types of research, the two main higher degrees in the United Kingdom are the MD and PhD. The PhD can be undertaken by all scientists from both clinical and non-clinical backgrounds, whereas the MD is aimed at people with a medical background.

- In general, the MD is less structured and requires less formal supervision and can sometimes be undertaken on a part-time basis, for example while still maintaining clinical duties. This may be as a series of projects or papers. The MD requires a thesis to be written up, and there is a subsequent viva that has to be passed. Some universities may simply require a portfolio of publications to be put together to be taken forward as an MD rather than a primary research project per se.
- A PhD generally (but not always) requires a greater time commitment and work, as well as more breadth of work and more formal supervision.

For both higher degrees, universities often require certain courses to be undertaken and may have a transfer examination at the halfway point. Undertaking a more formal research degree requires a substantial amount of work and it is therefore important to make sure you have a full understanding of the commitment and discipline needed. This can be gained from speaking to people who are currently undertaking such work or those who have completed similar projects.

Getting the deanery to support a period in research

Once you have found the correct institution and an appropriate supervisor and research project, the next step is to ask for permission from your deanery. This may be in the form of a one-year fellowship, which is often offered by a university in the first instance. If this is the case, you may simply need to request a one-year out-of-programme experience (OOPE), and this can be extended should your one-year turn into an MD or PhD.

The application process can take a long time and, like getting into research itself, requires a lot of forward planning. You should meet your academic supervisor and the regional programme director at the deanery either at your Record of In-training Assessment (RITA) or Annual Review of Competence Progression (ARCP), or in a less formal setting. Try to approach them early and give them a full outline of why you want to pursue research, and the opportunities available to you. You will often find that deanery officials are supportive of you going into research, especially if you have a well thought out plan and an offer from a good place in which to do your research. It may be helpful to enlist a consultant that you have recently worked with who knows you well and will be willing to write a letter to the deanery on your behalf supporting your time out of programme.

The process of applying for an OOPE, getting your postgraduate dean to sign off on this and coordinating this with your clinical attachments can take a long time. It is advisable to get the ball rolling 12 months before you want to start your research. You will still need to attend your yearly education assessments (ARCPs/RITAs) whilst in research, and you may need to also attend teaching/training sessions during this time, either within your deanery or at your new institution. You also need to keep up to date with clinical skills and show this in a formal way. This will depend very much on your deanery as well as on your own specialty; for example, surgical trainees may need to attend skills teaching sessions or maintain anatomy teaching commitments.

Clinical duties during research

Once you get into research, especially if it is full time, you need to decide whether you want or need to pursue some clinical duties too. This may be needed in terms of funding. For example, it may be that your research post is funded partly through a university and partly through the NHS, requiring you to do a number of clinical sessions (e.g. perform on-call or clinic duties).

However, if the research is fully funded, it is important to decide whether you want to spend time in clinical medicine. This may be an advantage – for example if you need to collect clinical samples or if you want to maintain your clinical skills set. It may also give you the opportunity to work and make contacts in a very specialised setting – if you are researching a rare disease you may want to work in the outpatient setting for that condition. However, the downside of this is that the clinical work may take you away from your research. Spending one afternoon a week in the clinic may not seem much; but when you add in the dictation of clinic letters, attending the radiology and multidisciplinary team meetings, the follow-up of results and consultation with clinical colleagues, what on paper seemed like half a day in reality becomes much more. For these reasons, it is absolutely vital that, if you decide to do clinical work, you limit it as much as possible. After all, your time in research may be the only time you will ever have to get away from seeing patients.

More about funding

There are a number of ways of funding your research. They range from getting no money at all, to getting a fully funded research fellowship with one of the main research bodies. If you are very keen to pursue a research career and have not been able to get any funding, it may be that you can find a little bit of 'soft' money – a small pot of money available from a university to do your work while you do locums in your spare time. This can be very demanding of your time and your bank balance, but for those who have no other option it may be the only way to get into research. After a short period you may be able to apply for some funding to allow you to continue the research, based on your preliminary results.

Clinical fellowships

Funding often comes directly from a university or other academic institution. This may be for an initial 12 months, and there are advertisements in journals such as the *British Medical Journal* for these posts. The advertisement may state that a 12-month clinical fellow position is available for a specific project and that this could be extended for 2–3 years towards a higher degree.

It is important to think carefully about these positions, because sometimes the funding may run out after the initial 12 months. You should go and meet with the potential supervisor to discuss the exact economics of the position before applying. If they admit that they have only 12 months' worth of funding at this point, ask do you want to spend a year of your life on a particular project with the real risk that there might be no further money to continue the work? If it is in an exciting area then you might consider the risk worth taking, or simply go into the project feeling that the skills you gain will allow you to continue academic work elsewhere if necessary.

The money might be available for the full 2–3 years for the right applicant, in which case these positions become far more desirable. They may be very competitive, but will allow you to register for a higher degree up front and you will be secure in the knowledge that your funding is in place.

Similar positions may be available from individual academics who have large project grants from which they can pay a researcher's salary. Again, these positions are more competitive but far more desirable than a post with only 12 months of funding.

Research training fellowships

Personal fellowships become available from organisations such as the Medical Research Council, the Wellcome Trust or the National Institute of Health Research. These are the most competitive forms of funding as they allow clinicians to pursue a research project of their own choice, rather than have to work on a stipulated project. The awards are made to universities to give out, or can be applied for directly from the funding bodies. The latter form of application needs to be made several months in advance of a start date and requires a great deal of work and planning.

Writing a successful fellowship proposal for yourself can be very daunting, especially if you have no background in grant writing. It is vital that you choose the right project, the right place and right person to supervise you, and that you are the best candidate. These three things – Project, Place, Person – constitute the three 'P's and are the most important aspects of your proposal that grant bodies are looking for. As long as you can show you have a certain level of enthusiasm and intelligence, you do not necessarily have to be well published or have a lot of research experience in order to get a fellowship. More important is the place, supervisor and project that you want to do. Working with a supervisor of the highest class can take you from being an enthusiastic clinician towards being a serious clinical academic – and that is what grant bodies are looking for.

Writing a successful grant application takes effort. You first have to find a supervisor who is willing to support your application and supervise you for the duration of the research. The person has to be willing to help you write the grant application, so it is important that your supervisor(s) has a good track record with similar grant bodies. Once you have found such a supervisor who is willing to take you on, you need to choose an area of interest. This must be something that you yourself feel very passionate about, and that the supervisor is familiar with. The idea itself has to be exciting and innovative but should not be too ambitious, as the grant body wants to ensure that you can achieve much of what you are asking to do in the allocated time.

When deciding the project itself and the type of work involved, spend time within the group to get an understanding of the methods used and perhaps obtain some pilot data. If you are fortunate to be on an academic pathway (e.g. as an Academic Fellow), then this may be performed as part of your clinical rotation. If not, then you may have to work even harder and spend your free time in the group to try to generate some data which supports your idea. In fact, if you have had to do this in your spare time, it often looks far better to a grant body.

Once you have decided on a project, you will have to compose a 'lay' summary and a scientific summary.

- The lay summary has to explain your work in a very straightforward but not overtly simple way, such that a non-medical member of the public can understand the thinking behind your proposal.
- The scientific summary has to outline the scientific/clinical basis for the concept of your study.

Both can be very difficult to summarise in a few hundred words, so write several drafts with your supervisor before you submit the final version.

You will have to detail your full clinical career to date, any previous publications, and your desire for a career in academic research. Several pages will then be devoted to the actual structure of the project – you will have to lay out why your study idea is feasible and achievable, and what impact it will have on medicine as a whole.

The last part of the form is usually about the financial aspects and this can take a long time to sort out. It must be done in conjunction with the university's financial departments. You will have to generate a range of figures, including your own salary, costs of consumables and other scientific expenditures, patient recruitment, sample storage, travel to meetings etc. On average, it costs approximately (in current terms) £100 000 to perform a year of clinical research, so a three-year PhD project might cost in the region of £300 000. This large amount of money takes into account your salary, all university overheads, the cost of part of your supervisor's time, and any equipment that you use, for example in the laboratory.

Your research salary will usually be calculated as an unbanded post and, although it will be a drop from a full clinical salary, it is much greater than the salary of a typical research student.

Applications will have to be submitted by the university by a particular deadline. Details of these can be found at the relevant websites (see below), but the process itself takes several months. There may be an initial application, a full application, and then if successful, an interview. At the interview stage, it is vital that you have well-versed answers for a range of questions that frequently arise. The interview normally takes around half an hour. The panel is composed of between 10 and 15 clinical academics as well as basic science researchers. They often spend just a few minutes on your own clinical background and then spend the majority of the time on your hypothesis. You must know the exact details of the work involved, the background papers and publications, the techniques involved, and details of the ethics needed for the work.

You must also know what is achievable within your time frame so that the grant bodies know that you have a realistic plan. Grant bodies make grants to clinicians within the hospital and general practice, as well as to other clinicans such as vets and clinical psychologists. It is therefore important that you have a good plan for your own future academic clinical career when you sit down in any interview. The rejection rate is high, so be prepared to apply to multiple grant bodies at the same time, something you need to explain in each application.

In addition to the three main UK-based research organisations covered in the following sections, there are a number of other large funding bodies, and these are often disease- or system-specific. Some offer grants and project money. Please consult the (non-exhaustive) list at the end of this chapter.

The Medical Research Council

The MRC traces its origins to the Royal Commission Appointed to Inquire into the Relations of Human and Animal Tuberculosis, which was set up in 1901. In 2008/9 the MRC spent £758 million on medical research and provided a range of junior and senior funding as well as project grants.

Specifically, for those starting out in research, there is the Clinical Research Training Fellowship, which is advertised three times a year. The fellowship:

> provides up to three years' support for clinically qualified, active professionals to undertake specialised or further research training in the bio-medical sciences within the UK. A further year's funding is available for patient-orientated clinical research training fellowships. The scheme is designed to accommodate the dual clinical–research training career path by allowing fellows to spend up to 20 per cent of their time on NHS sessions. Fellows are required to register for a research degree, normally a PhD, based on research undertaken during the fellowship.

The Wellcome Trust

The Wellcome Trust was founded by Sir Henry Wellcome (1853–1936), an American businessman and philanthropist who came to consolidate his business empire in the UK. In 2010 the trust had a total fund worth of over £12 billion. It funds a number of fellowships and project grants, but specifically for junior clinicians it funds the Research Training Fellowships which are advertised three times a year:

> This scheme is for medical, dental, veterinary or clinical psychology graduates who have little or no research training, but who wish to develop a long-term career in academic medicine. Applications are encouraged from individuals who wish to undertake substantial training through high-quality research in an appropriate unit or clinical research facility, towards a PhD or MD qualification. Fellowships are normally for two to three years. In exceptional cases a fellowship may be for up to four years for those who wish to undertake a relevant Masters training or diploma course. All training requests must be fully justified in the application. Fellowships provide research expenses (consumables, travel, support to attend scientific meetings, fieldwork and data collection) and a fellow's salary, set according to age, experience and our policy on enhancement. The necessary equipment and facilities required for the proposed research must be available to the candidate, so it is essential that a laboratory or unit appropriate to the research proposed is selected. Substantial requests for equipment are not accepted.

The National Institute of Health Research

This is a UK government body responsible for research within the NHS. Its mission statement is: 'improving the health and wealth of the nation through research'. It funds a number of fellowships and project grants, but specifically for junior clinicians it funds the Doctoral Research Fellowships which are advertised once a year:

> *The Doctoral Research Fellowship (NIHR-DRF) offers three years of full-time funding (or four or five years part-time) to undertake a PhD and is aimed at individuals, of outstanding potential, early in their research careers. It aims to fast-track them through a customised research training programme in an environment reflecting their individual talents and training needs. It is anticipated that successful applicants would become independent research leaders within 6–10 years of completing an NIHR-DRF award.*

Sources of further information

Alzheimer's Association: www.alz.org/research/overview.asp

British Heart Foundation: www.bhf.org.uk

British Lung Foundation: www.lunguk.org

Cancer Research UK: www.cancerresearchuk.org

Medical Research Council: www.mrc.ac.uk

National Institute of Health Research: www.nihr.ac.uk/research/Pages/default.aspx

Research Councils UK: www.rcuk.ac.uk

Royal Society: http://royalsociety.org/grants

UK Clinical Research Collaboration: www.ukcrc.org

Wellcome Trust: www.wellcome.ac.uk

8

Research: getting results

Key aims of this chapter

- Give an overview of the key aims of research
- Discuss the best approach to writing up and finishing research
- Explore the decisions around continuing research.

Introduction

Starting a project within a well-established research group can be daunting, especially if you are new to the concept of research. Working in a large group of individuals with different skills and personalities is always difficult. It is therefore important from the outset that you understand your own aims for your time out of clinical practice. On the flip side, it can be very exciting to be thrust into a new environment where you get to meet dedicated scientists at the top of their game who are passionate about the work they do.

Starting research

Administration

Ensure that you have filled in all the necessary paperwork for your research degree. This will include registration forms from the university which detail your type of work, degree and timescale for finishing the work. You may also be asked to select examiners for your halfway (upgrade) viva at the very beginning, and it is important that you choose these carefully with input from your supervisor. They should ideally be academics in your field who will give you a careful and thorough examination, but not at the expense of demeaning your work.

At the outset of your research project you may be asked to sign up to courses that are required for your degree. Make sure you have completed the correct number of these by the time you finish. You may also be asked to sign up for journal clubs, departmental presentations and other academic rotas. If your work involves clinical samples or patients, you may have to apply for ethics to do the studies both within a hospital or within a local region. You may need to apply for honorary contracts in new hospitals to see patients, and these will require substantial paperwork of their own.

In addition to research administration, you may need to complete some paperwork from your deanery. If your research time is being taken as an out-of-programme (OOP) experience, you will need to keep in touch with the deanery on a regular basis and you may have to keep a record of your teaching attendance. Additionally, if you are in a surgical specialty you may have to show evidence of ongoing skills competency. Finally, if you want to extend your time out of programme then you will need to inform your deanery and get permission well in advance.

Hypotheses and plans

Any research project will need a strong hypothesis and set of aims. This is applicable equally to laboratory science as it is to patient-based clinical research. The importance of having a strong hypothesis is that it allows you to have a benchmark to test your ideas against. Well thought out plans will help you achieve your research aims. Having said this, it is extremely likely that parts of your research project will have to be changed during your project because research never goes exactly to plan. Results, difficulties and changes to methodology along the way will alter your plans, while not necessarily altering the overall scope of your work. Have a back-up plan in case the main project does not go entirely as expected.

As part of this process, review your work on a regular basis with your supervisor as well as with other members of the research team. This will help you track your progress and check whether you are heading towards your goals. It will additionally enable you to make any needed changes before it becomes too late. It may also help to have an external review of your work from researchers outside the group. However, if you plan on discussing your results with outside members, get approval and support from your supervisor first.

Occasionally, research projects completely falter. It could be that the project was unworkable, the methods were unsuccessful, or outside factors were at play (e.g. personal circumstances made the ongoing project difficult). It is important to identify such problems early, to give you and the university time to make alternative plans. These may include terminating the research project, leaving early with an alternative degree (e.g. an MA instead of an MD), or moving to a completely new project or research group for the remainder of your time. In such cases, it is not at all unusual for the university to step in and assist as they will have dealt with many such instances before.

Supervision

All research requires supervision. For a formal research degree such as an MD or PhD, there will be a named supervisor. He or she will have the responsibility of seeing your project through from start to finish and ensuring that you receive good scientific training along the way.

Use your supervisor's time and advice wisely, particularly if he or she has more than one student. The supervisor might be hard to pin down, or might seem more interested in other people's work rather than your own; and even when the supervisor does sit down with you, you might not receive all the supervision you require. This is a common scenario in clinical academia where people have to juggle science, clinical duties, teaching and partnerships with industry, leaving them less time to supervise students. It can be a difficult problem, especially if your supervisor was solely responsible for you starting research in the first place, but there are a number of tactics you can use to get adequate supervision.

First, try to arrange regular supervisory meetings. Your university timetable may stipulate that you have a minimum number of supervisions per quarter, but even if it does it is important to have an additional regular set of meetings. This may be once a week or once a month; but whatever the frequency, the meetings must be just for you and your supervisor to discuss your ongoing work. Try to make sure there are minimal interruptions and, if things are not working out, suggest an alternative time of day to meet or even an alternative location away from your research institute (e.g. the local coffee house) to make sure you have dedicated research time. If this doesn't work, then try to explain in writing (in the form of emails) that you feel that the meetings are not working and that your supervisor needs to suggest alternative methods of discussing your work.

If this does not help and you have another supervisor, then try to get him or her involved at the same time. It may be helpful to arrange joint supervision meetings, or at least play supervisors off against each other by extolling their virtues in joint emails. It may be helpful to find alternative informal supervision from members outside your research group but, again, it is important that you inform your own supervisor before making such arrangements.

Finally, there is a process of formal reporting for both MDs and PhDs and this involves reports to the university detailing ongoing supervision. It is mandatory in the UK that part of this reporting is directly from the students to the university, bypassing the supervisors. This may be the best opportunity to explain the shortcomings in your research supervision, but it is helpful to confront a lacklustre supervisor prior to reporting any problems in writing. Notwithstanding, if you feel there is a problem it is important that you report it sooner rather than later.

Mentorship

Mentors are different from supervisors. The Academy of Medical Sciences (see links at the end of this chapter) has a formal mentorship scheme and this can be accessed by researchers looking for formal guidance. They describe mentorship as:

> *essentially about helping people to help themselves and is most commonly used to describe the (formal or informal) process whereby an experienced person (the mentor) guides another individual (the mentee) in their personal, professional development.*

In any research project it is vital that you find one or more mentors to see you through your work. They should ideally be unrelated to your supervisor so that they can give you an objective view on your own work. It may also be helpful if they are outside your exact sphere of work, again to be able to give their own perspective on your work. Mentors can give you academic as well as personal advice and should fully understand your future career aspirations.

Mentors can be research based or purely clinical. It may even be helpful to have multiple mentors to fulfill different aspects of your own learning needs. Mentorship can be formal in some situations. For example, some universities require a named mentor on all project outlines in addition to a named supervisor. Mentors can also be informal, and in such cases they can be sought out through your own research department. You may be able to find retired academics who are willing to spend time guiding you. Alternatively, you may be able to find mentors by speaking to clinicians with whom you have worked previously.

Daily research life

It can be helpful to keep a diary or journal of your time in research. This will give you an overview and is a tool used by many clinicians to show them an overall plan of their work. However, in addition, it is important that you keep notes of your research on a regular basis. Then you can go back and review your work and make sure that the data you have collected or results you have generated are as reproducible as possible. Many people make handwritten notes but it can be helpful to type these up as you go along. An electronic version of your research notes can be quickly copied and backed up, as well as shared easily with the appropriate people.

Your working times in research are likely to be very different from what you are used to in the clinical world. Most clinicians in research will find that they are able to come and go as they wish. Laboratory work requires timed experiments and these may keep you working late or need you to start early. You can offset this by changing your start or finish times in the laboratory. Collecting clinical samples from an afternoon clinic that then need processing until the early evening may mean that you come in late the next day. Analysis of data or writing-up of results can often be done at home with access to the appropriate software on your own computer or through the university intranet. Most supervisors will be happy for you to dictate your own working times as long as you make good progress.

In addition to your own work, there will be ample opportunity for furthering your knowledge. If your research is directly attached to a university there will be facilities for journal clubs, departmental meetings, internal and external lectures. Try to make the most of these opportunities to improve your knowledge in your own area as well as in related fields. For example, if your research is in genetics of malaria infection you may be able to attend lectures on genetic analysis techniques, clinical updates in malaria and epidemiology of infectious diseases. Attending lectures by members outside of your direct research department will allow you to discuss your own work with others in the field as well as build up new contacts to help with your current and any future work.

You may need to participate in some clinical work as part of your research funding. If not, you may be asked to do some clinical work in addition to your research work. However, it is essential that you limit your clinical work to what is vital for your own research and specialist training, rather than simply providing a clinical service to a hospital with no benefit to your ongoing research.

Managing your finances

Research salaries are invariably less than when in clinical training. It is important to ensure that your salary is taxed appropriately at this level. The best funded posts are essentially paid at an unbanded level, but this can be topped up with locum clinics and on-calls as needed – see Chapter 7. These posts are usually placed under the umbrella of university staff and you may not be eligible for any student amenities. However, if you are classed as a student you may be eligible for discounts on council tax and train fares, for instance. Contact your university finance office as soon as you start research to clarify your position. Importantly, staff do not need to pay tuition fees whereas students may have to.

In addition to your own personal finances, you may be asked to manage your research finances. If you have your own grant then you will have access to be able to order consumables and research equipment without approval. If not, you may be asked in some instances to get approval from your supervisor before purchasing items such as expensive pieces of equipment. You should be able to get regular information from your department finance officer as to the overall state of your funding so that you can spend or save money as appropriate. There may also be money available for conferences and travel.

Keeping up to date

You must keep up to date with changes in your research area and in your own clinical specialty. Keeping abreast of research advances will require regular journal reading and online searches for new publications. You will need to talk to people both inside and outside your department who are working in the same area. By attending the relevant meetings and conferences you may also be able to find out about unpublished or soon-to-be-published advances that directly affect your research.

Keeping up to date with your clinical field is as important. This is especially true for those researchers who have left clinical medicine completely for an extended period. You will need to read up on advances in your area and attend deanery and hospital teaching sessions. Registering for clinical specialist meetings may also be helpful to be aware of recent changes to basic clinical management. Alternatively, simply catching up with clinical colleagues in a social setting should help you keep one foot in the clinical world as you pursue your research project.

Writing it up

Your thesis

An MD or PhD will require a formal thesis to be written up and presented to the university as evidence of your research project. This work does *not* have to summarise everything you attempted; it *does* have to be a concise and scientifically written account of your findings.

Obtain some examples of previously written projects, which should be available for your reading in your department. There might be a particular style that has to be adhered to. This will include a maximum word count, information on how to present tables or figures, and the general layout of chapters. Most research reports start with a background chapter and then a methods chapter before moving into results. The conclusions can be written at the end of each chapter or as a separate chapter at the end. Again, it is important to review previous examples before writing your own thesis. References will have to be written carefully, a task that will be made considerably easier by using one of the available electronic reference programs.

A thesis is a published document that is kept within the university, so it must be as accurate and truthful as possible. Universities use software to detect plagiarism, so it is paramount that the work is your own only. It is also possible to plagiarise your own work (e.g. by inserting text from a publication that you have written into your thesis). Check with the university for the exact rules regarding this.

You may find it best to start writing the background chapter long before your deadline for handing in the thesis. This can be modified as you progress, but will form a strong starting point from which to continue writing. Most people take off a period of time to write their thesis either in the library or at home. This process can take several months, depending on the amount of data you have to present, and so should not be underestimated.

Aim to have your writing finished before you leave research and return to the clinical world. You will find it much harder to write the thesis once you

are back dealing with patients full time. The longer you leave it, the less
likely you are to complete the task.

Handing in your thesis and attending the viva

Make sure you have followed the correct administration procedures according to the university guidelines. Most universities require notice before you submit so that they can get their own systems in place. They will need to have appointed examiners (chosen by you and your supervisor) prior to you submitting the thesis. Typically there will be one internal examiner who is there to make sure that the proceedings are fair and balanced, and one external examiner to interrogate the thesis. However, in some cases there may be several examiners and some universities allow your supervisor (or even other members of the research group) to sit in.

The thesis will have to be handed in to the university, either printed or in electronic format for them to print. The university will then send off viva copies directly to the examiners. These are cheaper paper copies for them (and you) to make notes on. You will have to take one copy to the viva. The viva may not take place until several months after you submit your thesis.

The viva itself is often an anticlimax. Despite the examiners having read your thesis, it is inevitable that you will know more about the subject than them. Your examiners may wish to hurry up the process and, if they are generally happy with the work, the entire process may be very short – less than an hour or two. However, in some cases it can be much longer.

Most universities have a simple system of scoring. The unlikely scenarios are that the exam is passed immediately (as there will always be queries with the thesis) or that it is failed (as your supervisor is unlikely to allow you to sit the viva if there is a possibility you could fail). Much more likely are minor corrections (e.g. spellings, visualisation of tables or charts) or major corrections (e.g. more laboratory experiments or further data analysis). In such cases you will have a set amount of time to complete these corrections and return them to the examiners before the degree can be passed and your final thesis copies printed off.

Wider publication of your results

You should attempt to have your research published in peer-reviewed journals. It is possible to publish one piece of work that encompasses your research project, but those who are hardworking (and lucky) may be able to publish more. In addition, there may be an opportunity to publish book chapters or reviews. Moreover, it may also be possible to collaborate with other groups (e.g. allow them use of your equipment or clinical samples) and this may lead to a publication. Finally, it is important that you are acknowledged in any future work that builds upon your research project. This may be in the form of an authorship on a research paper if appropriate.

What next?

Getting back into clinical work

Before returning to clinical work it will be vital to be fully prepared. This is especially important if your research has not been clinical and you have been effectively out of clinical practice for a number of years. Speak to colleagues in your next clinical attachment to find out exactly what your responsibilities will be. For example, if you are a medical registrar returning to hospital after three or four years in laboratory work it will be helpful to ascertain exactly which medical procedures you will be responsible for; you might have to place intercostal chest drains out of hours or it may be that there is a dedicated chest registrar at night to do this for you.

It can be helpful to go on courses to refresh your clinical training. This might include an advanced life support course, those dealing with practical procedures, or those involving diagnostic techniques, such as a refresher course on reading ECGs. For those in surgical training there may be a need to keep your skills logbook up to date during research, and you may need to show evidence of this in any new position.

Keeping a hand in research

Regardless of whether you wish to pursue an academic career, keep in touch with your research group once you have left. This will allow you to finish off any work that you may wish to do (e.g. you may be able to return on an ad hoc basis to complete laboratory work needed for a specific publication). It also means that you will be remembered by your research group as you continue in the clinical world – which will make it easier for them to put your name on a paper or recommend you for further research positions should you wish to pursue them. There may also be funding from your group for your travel back to the department or even for you to attend courses, lectures or conferences once you have left.

Choosing an academic career

The decision to pursue an academic career after you have carried out a period of research is a difficult one. The advantages to such a career include the ability to perform potentially ground-breaking science, the potential to lead and manage a group, and the freedom from clinical duties that come with a research position. This includes the fact that senior clinical researchers will be able to manage much of their own time and devote part of their working week to teaching, management or influencing public policy. For those who are successful there may also be added financial rewards such as NHS awards and links with pharmaceutical or biotechnology companies.

However, there are a number of disadvantages with an academic career. These include the constant pressure to perform by attracting research grants and publishing in peer-reviewed journals. The politics between senior clinical researchers is often fraught with more difficulties than that seen with senior clinicians. There is reduced scope for private practice, and an important drawback is the reduction in direct clinical interaction with both colleagues and patients. However, for those who are interested in pursuing an academic career, there are numerous options as outlined below.

- *Clinical lecturer posts*. These are not appointed through a university but through the relevant deanery. They are at an ST level and allow for a division of research and clinical work, often 50 per cent in each sphere. However, they do not attract research money, so this needs to be applied for in addition to the post itself.
- *Post-doctoral fellowships and intermediate funding*. These are relatively prestigious methods of funding and require a strong track record with a clear aptitude for academic work. They are available from organisations such as the Medical Research Council and the Wellcome Trust. They allow for dedicated research time outside of clinical work (e.g. two years of research work as time out of programme) and include money for research as well as funds to travel and attend conferences.
- *Senior lecturer posts*. These are usually appointed at a consultant level through a university. As with clinical lecturer posts (see above), they allow for time to be split between clinical work and research but also require long-term funding from other sources for associated research costs.
- *Senior funding and project grants*. These are available from the same places as intermediate funding (see above). They are often made to

clinical academics at the highest level and are for long periods (e.g. 5 years). They may pay an entire salary, allowing you to perform clinical duties as needed. They will also pay for support staff, research students, equipment and consumables.

Sources of further information

Academy of Medical Sciences: www.acmedsci.ac.uk

Cancer Research UK: www.cancerresearchuk.org

Medical Research Council: www.mrc.ac.uk

National Institute for Heath Research (NIHR): www.nihr.ac.uk/research

Research Councils UK: www.rcuk.ac.uk

The Royal Society: http://royalsociety.org/grants

UK Clinical Research Collaboration: www.ukcrc.org

Wellcome Trust: www.wellcome.ac.uk

9

Teaching

Key aims of this chapter

- Give an overview of the different types of teaching
- Provide tips on dealing with difficult teaching situations
- Outline courses and qualifications.

Introduction

Knowledge exists in two forms – lifeless, stored in books, and alive, in the consciousness of men.

(Albert Einstein, 1954)

Teaching others is a skill that appears inherent to clinicians. Throughout our medical school and postgraduate years we are constantly learning and building upon our knowledge as new evidence is found and new techniques are developed for the management of patients. This process of learning takes place in a vast number of arenas and formats, from sitting in a didactic neuroanatomy lecture as a medical student to, as a consultant neurosurgeon, learning new operative skills from a more learned collea-gue. Just as people learn at different paces, the skill to teach others comes more naturally to some doctors than to others.

In this chapter we look at types of teaching and what situations to use them in. We also discuss when it is appropriate to teach and how to balance this with your daily clinical commitments. Finally, we discuss the courses and qualifications available to develop their teaching skills.

Kolb's teaching styles

With all forms of teaching there is a particular style that can be adapted to the environment. There are many methods of detailing this, but one of the most popular is from David Kolb, an American teacher who published his learning styles model in 1984 with the proposition that 'learning is the process whereby knowledge is created through the transformation of experience'. Simply put, the style involves a series of four steps to allow students to learn effectively:

1 *Concrete experience.* The teacher explains a new experience or details a new interpretation of an existing experience, such as a new method of performing a lumbar puncture that is a slight variation on an accepted method.
2 *Reflective observation.* The concrete experience is reflected upon, perhaps through discussion of the differences between the old and new methods.
3 *Abstract conceptualisation.* After reflection, this is the idea of conceptualising the new method and deciding when it can be used.
4 *Active experimentation.* The student tries out the new technique for lumbar puncture and decides whether it is indeed better than the old method.

Rather than appearing as a straightforward progressive list, these four stages are actually applicable to different styles of learning by different students. This is something that needs to be taken into account in any teaching situation. The four styles are typically represented by four types of people – those who feel, watch, think or do:

- *Concrete experience.* These students like to evaluate their feeling about a learning point (e.g. examining their thoughts about whether a new way of performing a lumbar puncture is better than the old method).
- *Reflective observation.* These students like watching a learning point (e.g. watching the new lumbar puncture technique as a way of learning about it).
- *Abstract conceptualisation.* These students like thinking about a learning point (e.g. being taught about the new procedure and investing some time thinking about how it could be an improvement on the traditionally accepted method).

- *Active experimentation*. These students like doing things for themselves (e.g. learning about a new procedure and simply getting out and applying it in the real world).

As you teach new students in the clinical setting it is useful to bear these different styles in mind to find out which type of learner each student is. This will allow you to play to their strengths and give them the best teaching experience possible.

Types of teaching

There are a number of types or styles of teaching that doctors can use in the clinical setting to teach others. All types have strengths and weaknesses and these are discussed below.

Bedside clinical teaching

Bedside teaching can be informal during ward rounds or on-calls, or can be formal – for example, when teaching medical students as part of their finals revision or junior doctors as part of their revision for specialist exams.

Bedside teaching has a number of advantages. It can be fun and interactive as well as providing an excellent teaching experience. However, in order to do it well, it has to be thoroughly planned out in advance and the teacher has to understand the topics well. For example, after examining a patient with a pleural effusion you need to be able to have a full discussion with the students about the causes, investigations and appropriate management.

When taking students to see a patient, a number of simple rules need to be followed.

Find suitable patients

- Ask your colleagues for good cases in the hospital or GP setting in advance, rather than keeping a tutor group waiting while you struggle to find a willing or suitable candidate.

Obtain verbal consent

- Explain to the patients that you are asking for help to teach more junior clinicians and that their refusal to help will in no way influence their clinical care.
- Ensure that you have asked the patient for permission in a confidential setting prior to bringing students to the bedside.

- Tell patients that you can do the teaching now or, if it is later, give them an approximate time and tell them that family members can be present if they wish.
- Make sure that curtains are closed or that the exam is carried out in a private setting.

Make the most of bedside teaching

- Limit the number of clinicians you take to the bedside to just a handful. This will allow for a better teaching experience and will be less intimidating to a patient.
- If you have a large group, you can limit the number who examine the patient. For example, only one student performs a full cardiovascular examination but all the others can listen over the appropriate area for the heart murmur.
- Make time at the end of each case to viva the students. Ask them to present their findings (much as they would in 'real life' to a senior colleague or in an exam) and plan a course of management.
- You may wish to viva one student at a time or divide up the viva session to ask each student a series of questions, thus ensuring that everyone participates, even the most shy students.
- After seeing the patient, ensure that every student thanks them for their cooperation.
- Ensure that sensitive discussions take place away from the bedside (e.g. when discussing a prognosis).

For more formal teachings sessions, plan your time wisely. It is better to review a few good cases well rather than try to pack too many into a session. Moreover, if you are planning a teaching rota for students or juniors, make sure that this is comprehensive and builds up to the big day. Ensure that you have covered all the major topics that are likely to come up, well before the exam. This may require you to use a number of teaching methods, from bedside examinations and vivas to quizzes and small group tutorials or case-based discussions.

Teaching on the job

Teaching on the job involves teaching students, juniors and nurses as you conduct your day-to-day clinical activities. It can be very easy to incorporate into your own work as well as help you improve your clinical skills and reinforce your clinical knowledge.

This form of teaching can be very variable. For example, it may be that as a GP partner you let a medical student sit in a surgery with you and watch you receive patients, while quizzing the student in between seeing the patients and allowing him or her to examine interesting cases. Another example is a gastroenterologist teaching her specialist trainee how to perform an endoscopy. This form of passive learning can be easily incorporated into routine clinical care, but it has the disadvantage that, owing to time constraints, discussion of cases will be limited so you may be able to teach the salient points only.

For practical procedures, a common approach is 'see one, do one, teach one'. For example, when inserting a venflon it is possible to allow one medical student to first see you put one in, then do one himself or herself, before that student teaches others how to put a venflon in. For more complicated procedures it is advisable to take it in steps: allow your trainee to attempt different parts of the procedure (starting with the simplest) under supervision, and finally the whole procedure initially under supervision and then independently. Another possibility is to show your trainee the procedure being performed under different conditions first before attempting it unassisted. For example, when placing chest drains you can ask your junior to watch you place several drains in different anatomical positions for different indications, and then supervise the person placing several drains before allowing him or her to place them independently. Only after achieving this may they be competent at teaching others – although they would be in a position before this to describe the indications for the procedure and the procedure itself.

Ethical considerations are always important when teaching on the job. Permission needs to be gained from patients prior to teaching. For example, there could be a sign at clinic reception telling patients that medical students are present and that they should inform the receptionist if they wish to be seen by the doctor only. Even if consent is presumed in outpatients, it is important to let patients know that there is a student sitting in as soon as they walk through the door.

In terms of training junior doctors, this consent can be less explicit. Often it will be the specialist registrar or core trainee who obtains consent for a procedure that may or may not be performed under general anaesthesia or sedation. The operating surgeon may be the person obtaining consent (e.g. the registrar), and he or she should indicate this, or that they will be assisting or performing part of the procedure with the consultant in attendance. If the operating surgeon is not the person obtaining consent, he or she should, and usually will, have contact with the patient before the operation.

Teaching while on call

In the hospital setting, being on call can be a very useful time to teach others. As with all forms of teaching, the experience can be very varied – from a medical junior teaching medical students how to clerk inpatients on-call, to a surgical consultant quizzing her juniors on the post-take ward round.

The advantage of teaching when on call is that it offers a real life arena (which is often more memorable) within which to teach others. It can also help with the process of being on call. For example, asking students to see patients and initiate basic investigations before you review them can be a useful way of reducing your workload while also facilitating learning, as your students will feel more a part of the team. However, you should delegate tasks appropriately, according to the skill level of your student, since taking this approach could backfire and actually increase your workload (e.g. a student may order a series of unhelpful investigations which need to then be cancelled). A few simple tips can smooth the process of teaching when on call.

- Ensure that teaching is carried out during the quieter periods of an on-call – when there is adequate time for good teaching, though this may be unpredictable.
- Ask patients for permission. Let them know that a medical student may see them first and then present their findings to you before you review them yourself.
- Ensure that if more junior clinicians or students are seeing patients first, that appropriate patients are chosen (those with more stable conditions).
- If a patient is more unwell, then management can be carried out while a student reviews the patient more thoroughly. For example, you may take a brief history for a patient with a pneumothorax and ask a medical student to take a thorough and detailed history as you prepare for a chest drain insertion.
- Ensure that students are available for all practical procedures. For example, ask a junior to assist as you place a central venous line into a sick patient, and quiz the student about the anatomical landmarks as you do so.
- Encourage students to present a case in a more formal setting. For example, ask a medical student to present the history to the consultant on the post-take ward round.

- Remember, if things do become chaotic or stressful on call, this may not be an environment conducive to learning. You have a number of options, including: delegating your student to a specific related or unrelated task (e.g. asking the student to read about a topic and come and find you at a later stage); reallocating your student to a less busy colleague; or giving your student the option of going home.

Small group tutorials

This process involves teaching more than one student in a slightly more formal setting. Tutorials can be carried out with medical students, junior doctors, nurses, other healthcare staff or even with colleagues at the same level as you (e.g. a specialist trainee teaching other cardiology trainees on advanced echocardiography techniques). These tutorials can be informal or part of a teaching programme.

The advantage of such teaching is that it takes place within dedicated periods without interruption, and a number of different topics can be covered in each session in a structured manner. The main disadvantage is that, unlike on-call or on-the-job teaching, it requires planning in advance in order for the teaching sessions to be productive.

- Ensure that tutorials start and finish on time and let students know these times well in advance, in addition to any expected 'homework'.
- Find a quiet area or book a dedicated teaching room for the sessions.
- Make sure that students are clear about the aims and objectives of each teaching session at the start, and the 'ground rules'.
- Make the sessions as interactive as possible. For example, if reviewing examples of radiology, ask students to point out the abnormalities in a systematic manner.
- Encourage students to ask questions throughout the session and stimulate debate.
- Ensure that all the students participate.
- Allow the subject to be wide but be careful not to drift off topic.
- Begin each session with learning objectives and review these.
- At the end of the teaching session ensure that all the aims and objectives have been met (Box 9.1).

Seminars

These are similar to small group tutorials in terms of the method of preparation, aims and outcomes. However, the term is more commonly used

No matter what type of teaching you are involved with, it is always advisable to plan it in advance (unless it is an ad hoc teaching session). This need not take much time and you may be able to share lesson plans among different types of teaching. However, even a little effort will improve the experience for both you and your students.

- Have a set of objectives.
- Decide the content of your lesson and ensure these meet the objectives.
- Plan the order in which you will teach your session.
- Decide the methods of teaching – these may differ for the various parts of the lesson (e.g. reading out a list compared to role play).
- Make a point to review the objectives at the end of the lesson to see whether they have been met.
- Allow for questions.
- Allow for feedback, both to the students and from them to you, in order to better plan your next lesson.

Box 9.1 Planning a lesson

to describe teaching to peers that may occur over, for example, an entire day, covering one particular topic – such as urological cancers. Seminars can happen within a hospital setting (e.g. the postgraduate medical centre) or within a deanery (e.g. a deanery teaching day for all trainees in a particular specialty). It may be possible for you to get involved in the day's design, or in teaching as you become a more senior clinician. As a trainee, you could be involved if presentations from more junior members of the specialty are required; or it may be possible to assist in helping prepare these sessions by inviting speakers and helping to put together talks.

These opportunities are there to be had, so it is important that you find out what is available for you to get involved with.

Lectures

Lectures are more formal types of teaching. It is unlikely that you will be in a position to give lectures as a more junior doctor unless you have a specialist knowledge – for example, if you have undertaken a higher research degree and developed expertise in a particular area or technique. However, as you become more experienced, there will be the opportunity to give lectures especially to medical students, so it is worthwhile keeping your eye open for opportunities. They may be in the form of clinically based lectures or more basic science lectures.

There may also be the opportunity to deliver lectures to nursing students and physiotherapists as part of their training. If this is something that appeals to you, then contact medical or nursing school offices to offer your services. You could also contact the organisers of the numerous finals revision courses that are currently in existence.

Problem-based learning

This form of learning was initiated at McMaster University in Canada in the 1960s. It is currently used by a number of medical schools in the UK and other countries, and teaching hospitals have adopted it as their preferred method of teaching.

The aim is to task a group of students with a particular problem and ask them to work together to solve it. This can be during the session or in between sessions. For example, at the end of a teaching session the teacher may decide that heart failure is to be discussed at the next session. He or she may then ask each student to prepare a summary on a different aspect of heart failure (e.g. genetics of the disease, epidemiology, symptoms, examination findings, management and prognosis). Each student then effectively will teach the group by presenting his or her new knowledge at the next session – thereby improving their own learning as well as teaching others.

The main criticism of this method of teaching is that it asks students to assimilate a potentially large amount of information in each session, which can be counterproductive to their overall learning experience. One way to overcome this objection is to limit the amount of information presented and taught at each session, as well as to ask students to provide written summaries for each other at each session.

Types of student

Doctors

A significant amount of your teaching will be of other doctors. These may be more junior, at your level, or even sometimes doctors who are more senior than you. In all cases it is important to pitch your teaching at the right level.

Make sure you know the experience of your audience because it is not helpful if you attempt to teach them skills they already have. If the doctors are at your own level or more senior, consider asking them what they want to learn or get out of a teaching session; this will ensure that the time is put to best use. Be careful in pitching your level of teaching. It is as unhelpful, for example, to teach FY1 doctors advances in echocardiography as it is to teach cardiology ST6 doctors the differential causes of chest pain.

Doctors can, of course, be very demanding students. They may feel that they know more than you, or that your content is incorrect or that they would like a second opinion. Teaching doctors is, therefore, a skill that you develop and is refined through experience.

Medical students

Medical students are attached to an increasing number of clinical sites. Gone are the days when they would spend time only at a single teaching hospital and become familiar with all the departments contained within. They now attend clinics in a range of hospitals and GP surgeries and have attachments in district general hospitals. This means that as a more senior doctor you will invariably come into contact with students on a fairly regular basis (unless you are in a specialty such as occupational medicine or are a GP in a very rural practice). It is important, therefore, that you understand student's needs and teach them appropriately.

- Find out whether the students have a syllabus they have to follow and teach from this. For example, students attached to a firm for 6 weeks may have a set of topics that have to be covered.
- Ask about any assessments they will need to undertake.
- Pitch your teaching at the appropriate level. For example, final-year medical students will need to have a much greater depth and breadth of knowledge than more junior students.
- Aim to teach all aspects of a condition. For example, if teaching students about atopic dermatitis then review the aetiology, clinical findings and management as well as taking them to see real-life cases.
- Avoid embarrassing a student in front of their peers. The days of ritual humiliation are long gone and there is a fine line between pushing at the boundaries of someone's knowledge and making them feel uncomfortable – it can be misconstrued as bullying, which is a serious allegation.

- Try to involve students as much as possible by, for example, asking them questions in turn rather than singling out individuals.
- Work towards a goal. For example, review specific skills needed for an upcoming objective structured clinical exam (OSCE).

Nurses

Teaching nurses can be challenging. Pitch your lessons at the right level. For example, it may be appropriate to discuss the science of non-invasive ventilation with respiratory nurses, but this might not be appropriate for more general medical nurses. Nurses may also be interested in the practical aspects of clinical practice. So, for example, it may be appropriate for a new orthopaedic ward nurse to sit in on a postoperative clinic or observe an operation so that he or she is able to answer questions a patient asks while on the ward.

As with medical students, nursing students will have a syllabus, so aim to follow this as well as tailoring teaching to any forthcoming exam.

Support medical staff

It is useful if your teaching is not exclusively directed to other doctors, but also encompasses other allied healthcare professionals, such as paramedics, anaesthetic assistants and healthcare assistants. Much of this may be through on-the-job teaching rather than formal teaching sessions. This teaching is often organised by senior hospital consultants or by senior GP trainers, but doctors at all levels can get involved with it.

Challenging scenarios

Disruptive students

Your teaching as a doctor will usually be to individuals who are keen to learn rather than those who are there because they have to be. However, you will occasionally have to teach less keen students. They may be generally difficult people, or have a reason for a sudden change in attitude (e.g. difficult personal circumstances that make them more disruptive). It is important to explore the reasons for their disruption in order to both improve their learning and minimise disruption for other students. In most circumstances, a quiet word may be enough to solve the issue.

- If a student is regularly late or wants to leave teaching sessions early, explain that you may not be able to sign the student off for the entire period of teaching unless he or she can be present for the entire sessions.
- Students who keep attending to their phone may also need talking to outside the teaching session to explain that their constant distractions may be affecting the learning experiences of others, while also being disrespectful to you.
- Students who appear less than interested need to be confronted about their lack of interaction. This could be because they find the taught material too easy, or alternatively they might be sitting back as a coping mechanism because they do not fully understand the topic and are scared to ask for more help.
- Students who talk too much can be dealt with by allowing a few minutes of discussion at the beginning of the session and then announcing that it is time to start the lesson, rather than starting teaching as soon as everyone has arrived.
- With a student who is continuously disruptive, discuss your concerns in private. Let the student know that you are genuinely worried, and that could be enough to improve the situation.
- If any problem persists, it might be necessary to escalate matters and discuss the problem with their Head of Year.

Bright students

Students at any level who are very bright can be difficult to teach. As well as being more able than their peers, they may even know more than you as the teacher. In such circumstances it is important that you are able to challenge the student appropriately while still engaging with others who are there to learn from you.

- Allow the student to be pushed as far as he or she wishes to be. For example, suggest extra reading material and ask the student to find out about items not in the teaching syllabus.
- Allow for some extra time before or after a teaching session to go over any advanced learning points.
- Admit if you are unsure about something and ask the student to find out and let you know. This is far more valuable to both the student and the teacher than trying to give an answer that has dubious accuracy.
- If there are several teaching sessions (e.g. as part of a medical student syllabus), then encourage a bright student to work on a particular

problem and explore it at each teaching session. For example, when teaching a group of students attached to an infectious diseases firm specialising in tuberculosis, you could ask one student to prepare thoughts on why the organism is so resistant to treatment worldwide, and then explore different aspects of this at each teaching session.

- Suggest that a bright student helps his or her peers at each session. This is an avenue that can be fraught with difficulties but may help both the bright student and others if used appropriately.

Less able students

Students who are less able than others may need more help and more time. It could be that they are just less able in your area of teaching rather than in all areas; but in all cases they should be treated respectfully and not made to feel different.

- Allow extra time for students who appear to be struggling. Ask them questions at the end of a teaching session to make sure they understand the topic.
- If appropriate, allow students to arrive at a teaching session slightly earlier than their peers in order to give them more time to grasp the concepts being discussed.
- Encourage less able students to actively teach their own peers. This will help reinforce their own learning as well as improve their confidence.
- Provide less able students with more teaching information than others. For example, if teaching a session on depression, provide them with a greater selection of published reviews on the topic.
- Encourage less able students to ask as many questions as possible by creating a learning atmosphere where questioning is commonplace.
- Start each teaching session with the more challenging topics and end with easier concepts. This will allow students of all abilities to know how the lesson is planned and allow them to be prepared.

Multidisciplinary teaching

Multidisciplinary teaching can be difficult to perform effectively. By trying to teach the same topic to people of different skills at the same time, you run the risk of not teaching anyone at all. However, a few simple techniques may make the process more useful and enjoyable for all.

- Have a general set of aims, but split students into different groups for the topic. For example, if aiming to teach about intubation in intensive care, set out the overall aims and then ask nursing students to investigate the equipment used, medical students to think about indications for intubation, and junior doctors to discuss among themselves the disadvantages of intubation.
- Build on problems together. For example, if teaching radiology, ask students to run through the basic anatomy of a CT scan and junior doctors to then take over and point out the abnormalities.
- Ask students to work together. For example, if teaching advanced resuscitation to a group, ask the doctors and nurses to run through the scenario together as they would in real life.

Courses and qualifications

Teaching the teachers

These courses are aimed at clinicians who teach others. They are usually two-day courses run by a number of companies across the UK. They will have continuing professional development (CPD) accreditation and, importantly, attendance on such courses often results in extra points when shortlisting for more senior positions such as consultant jobs. Despite being reasonably expensive, the courses are often limited in the number of places they offer, so they can be fully booked several months in advance.

The courses offer small group teaching, breakout sessions and learning by examples. In general they include:

- the theory behind educational models
- development of different teaching methods
- how to assess the different learning styles of students
- how to plan a teaching session
- how to develop learning objectives
- methods of assessment
- tips on dealing with difficult students
- creating a safe and welcoming learning environment
- how to develop presentation skills
- how to give effective feedback to students
- how to listen and when to ask questions.

Postgraduate teaching qualifications

For those clinicians who are very keen to develop their teaching skills there are a number of teaching courses to take and certificates to obtain. These include postgraduate certificates in education (PGCEs), diplomas in medical education, and masters degrees in medical education. Courses are offered by a number of universities in the UK and can be taken full time, part-time or by distance-learning.

Sources of further information

Association for the Study of Medical Education: www.asme.org.uk

Centre for Medical Education (Dundee): www.dundee.ac.uk/meded

General Medical Council education and training: www.gmc-uk.org/education/index.asp

Medical Education England: www.mee.nhs.uk

Royal Society of Medicine trainees: www.rsm.ac.uk/yf/index.php

10

Management

Key aims of this chapter

- Discuss management styles
- Describe characteristics of a good leader
- Discuss specific methods of managing your own team.

Introduction

Not every junior doctor will want to get involved in top-level management, but all will find themselves having to manage others at some stage. Whether it is discussing the rota with your fellow registrars to make it fair for everyone, or sitting on a junior doctors' committee in the hospital, or even being appointed as the local BMA representative – management of one kind or another will play a significant role in your career. Because of this, it is useful to establish some principles and rules to guide the way you interact with your colleagues. Managing may come easily to some but harder to others. Managing your team, your time and your life can be difficult and it is useful to have a structure to approach this.

Management

Five management styles

There are a number of different management styles in use in everyday situations. Doctors tend to work in teams (or at least try to) but can use these different techniques for different situations. The academics Robert

Tannenbaum and Warren Schmidt wrote a ground-breaking article in the 1957 edition of the Harvard Business Review outlining five main styles of management. There are a number of modern variations of this, but in essence these five styles remain applicable today. Each style has both its strengths and its weaknesses.

Autocratic management

These managers can be seen as dictators rather than team players. Typically, they make all the decisions themselves and ask their teams to simply carry out the instructions. There might be some freedom in how team members carry out specific tasks. Alternatively, there might be little or no freedom and all tasks have to be carried out exactly as asked. In medicine there is the stereotype of an old-fashioned hospital consultant who barks orders at his team and makes medical students tremble and nurses cry on ward rounds. The advantage is that tasks are carried out efficiently and rapidly. The drawbacks include low team morale and lack of initiative by team members.

Democratic management

In this style, team members are given a strong voice and their viewpoints may be taken into consideration in the final decision. This is not practicable in a number of cases in medicine; for example, a consultant surgeon would not routinely ask all members of the operating team for information on where to cut next! However, it can work in some situations. A surgical registrar on call who has a number of patients to see may ask his team of juniors who they each would like to see and then divide up the patients as requested. This has caveats, of course. A sick patient would not be given to the most junior member of the team to review first. The advantage of such a management style is that it allows members to have a strong say and feel that they are valued members of the team. The downside is that it can be a slow process and lead to ineffectual leadership at the top.

Bureaucratic management

This involves a lot of administration and all decisions have to be signed off by the appropriate chain of command. In medicine, this process may be applicable to some hospital managers who need to get all decisions signed off in advance by the appropriate senior manager. In clinical medicine it may be found in the outpatient setting where all patients seen by a junior doctor need to be reviewed at each consultation by a more senior doctor. The advantage of this style is that there is good evidence-based accountability when things go wrong. The main drawbacks are the lack of initiative by team members and the increased time needed for decisions to turn into actions.

Paternalistic management

In this style, the leader is concerned with the welfare of all team members and ensures they are happy in their roles. In medicine, this may be a senior GP checking on a daily basis that his more junior associates are happy and content with work and functioning efficiently. Another example is a consultant psychiatrist asking his juniors to take counselling sessions on a frequent basis to improve both their own welfare and subsequently that of their patients. The main advantage is that team members are valued and happy in their roles. The drawback is that this style may be taken too far and the wellbeing of team members begins to take priority over that of the work itself.

Laissez-faire management

This is a laid back style of management where the leader allows team members to take active roles in the discussion and decision-making process. An example is that of a medical registrar on call who allows all juniors to see their own patients and then reviews them only if requested or required. He or she may make little input (unless there is a strong need to), thereby allowing team members to take a lot of responsibility for their own decisions. The advantage is that it allows for a relaxed working atmosphere and gives team members a significant level of independence. The main disadvantage is the possible absence of guidance from the team leader, which might lead to dangerous mistakes if other members of the team do not ask for help when needed.

Management by walking around

In addition to Tannenbaum and Schmidt's five styles of management, there is a newer concept called 'management by walking around' (MWA). This concept relies heavily on the fact that managers may gain new insights by leaving their headquarters and proceeding to see how their team members work on a daily basis. The advantage is that they get to see exactly what problems their team encounter first hand, so can use that information in developing methods to tackle these issues. The disadvantage is that most hospital consultants would not want to spend a night on call in the hospital with junior members of their team!

Fifteen qualities of a good manager

As a junior doctor, there are a number of qualities you will be able to improve upon in order to become a better manager of your team. Examples of these, along with potential scenarios that can arise in medicine, are given below. It is important for you to try to develop your own management skills. Concentrate on areas where you feel you are weakest and improve these during your training, so you continually evolve.

1. Leadership

Aim to be a strong leader and someone to whom your team can look up for inspiration and advice. Think of an orthopaedic surgeon running two trauma calls simultaneously and asking all members of the team to work together in order to treat their patients as best as they can.

2. Communication

Communicate well both with members of your team and others around you. Think of dealing with a patient complaint against one of your junior staff members by allowing the patient and family to give their point of view and then communicating with them to ensure that further care is to the highest standard possible.

3. Organisation

Develop organisational skills to allow all the members of your team to be used in the most effective, appropriate and efficient manner. Think of a medical registrar running an on-call and allocating the team to see patients as competently and swiftly as possible.

4. Team morale

Improve the morale of your entire team with the aim of improving the output and quality of care. Think of a surgical consultant who buys coffee for the team on the post-take ward round while discussing the cases prior to going to see the patients.

5. Motivation

Motivate your team members to do the best they can. Think of a GP registrar who allows a foundation doctor attached to the practice to discuss his or her cases on a daily basis and encourages the junior to improve clinic skills during the course of his or her attachment.

6. Being a team player

Allow yourself to take a more subservient role if the situation calls for it. Think of a surgical registrar who allows her junior trainee to assist the consultant in an interesting operation rather than try to do it all herself.

7. Defining success

Explain to your team what measures of success you would want to use over a given period. Think of a renal consultant aiming to reduce the mean inpatient stay by one day over the course of 12 months through good multidisciplinary support.

8. Conflict resolution

Resolve problems among team members. Think of a dermatology registrar trying to sort out the rota with her colleagues and also dealing with any problems that arise between two foundation doctors over the allocation of leave.

9. Giving responsibility

Allow all team members to work to their capacity giving them further responsibility where appropriate. Think of allowing a junior doctor to perform a specific procedure unsupervised if you feel he has enough experience to do this by himself.

10. Taking responsibility

As a manager and a leader, take responsibility for your own mistakes and allow members of your team to see that you have done so. Think of a medical consultant who, having discharged a patient who then comes back into hospital almost immediately, explains to her team that she should have kept the patient on the ward for a little longer.

11. Holding people accountable

This involves telling members of your team if you feel that they are not up to the job and allowing them to be accountable. For example, ask your junior doctor to apologise to a family (with you in the room as appropriate) if he or she has made a significant error in patient care.

12. Time management

Insist on good time management for both yourself and members of your team. For example, ensure that post-take ward rounds do not overrun, causing the night team to have to stay longer than needed.

13. Mentorship

Act as a mentor to all members of your team. Think of a GP partner giving regular useful advice to trainees in her surgery about the obstacles to becoming a full partner and methods to overcome them.

14. Feedback

Give constructive criticism and feedback as appropriate. Think of a registrar pointing out both the good points and areas to work on to a medical student presenting a patient she has clerked when on call with the team.

15. Making people feel valued

Make all members of your team feel valued when they have done a good job. Think of a consultant on the post-take ward round who thanks the night team for looking after his on-call.

Managing your own team

Some problem areas

There are a number of management scenarios common to all specialties which you will need to be able to handle. These can arise at any stage of your career.

Juniors or colleagues who are late to work

This is a common scenario, especially when on call or working on a shift basis, such as in accident and emergency medicine. If you find that someone you work with is constantly late, the following may be useful.

- Confront the situation early. This is a better approach than leaving it for a long period before acting.
- Try to be consistent with all team members. Hold them all to the same standard in terms of punctuality and explain to those who are late that the standard is the same no matter the level of seniority.

- Ensure that there are no personal problems that are causing a consistent lateness and support or advise to help in any way with these issues (e.g. late night revision for exams or relationship problems).
- Explain that patients may suffer as a consequence of staff lateness. Give real examples where the team has suffered because of individuals not turning up on time.
- Give advice on how to organise his or her day better to turn up to work or shifts on time, but try not to be patronising, especially if the individual is having personal difficulties.

Doctors who lack motivation

As with those who are constantly late, this is a common scenario especially in jobs where fatigue has set in due to long and/or difficult working patterns (e.g. juniors in intensive-care medicine who do many nights and weekends). Personal problems may play a large role here, especially in junior doctors who are at difficult stages of their careers and may have multiple stresses such as exams, moving home, illness and financial strains.

- Try to offer as much support as possible if the individual is undergoing professional or personal difficulties. Explain that there will be many junior doctors in similar situations at that stage of their life.
- Try to find out what motivates the person. For example, if he has upcoming exams then discussing cases when on call in an exam format may help him improve his performance.
- Consider team-building exercises to integrate the individual better into the team and thereby improve his or her motivation (e.g. ensure that all the team can make a social event).
- If the person is really struggling, then ensure that he or she is aware of and directed towards appropriate professional resources of help (e.g. counselling).

Making mistakes

Everybody, doctors included, will make mistakes. When managing other members of staff who have made mistakes it is important that you support and guide them appropriately through the situation.

- Deal with the immediate consequences of the mistake first (e.g. urgent medical care) prior to any other actions.
- Ensure that there is full disclosure as appropriate. Small errors may only need to be discussed with a registrar, but a more serious error that

could lead to a complaint should be discussed with the most senior member of the medical team.

- Treat the error as a learning exercise and give constructive criticism and show how similar scenarios can be managed in the future.
- If the error is not an isolated event, try to see if there is something that can be done to avoid repetition. For example, a junior doctor who repeatedly causes problems when placing chest drains could be given more formal training and direct supervision when performing the procedure.
- Deal with complaints efficiently and fully. For example, if the family of a patient makes a complaint against a member of your team then ensure that this is dealt with in the correct manner in conjunction with the doctor against whom the complaint is made.

Nurturing your team

Managing a team of doctors and nurses is something that takes time and will improve with experience. There are a number of things you can do to improve team morale to obtain the best from team members. These are equally applicable to general practice as to hospital medicine and many of them are simply qualities that are found in any good team leader.

- Create a culture of openness and fairness where all team members are encouraged to discuss concerns and ways of improving patient outcomes.
- Have regular but brief meetings with your team during which everyone is encouraged to participate. Perhaps have a 5-minute meeting before ward rounds to discuss general ward issues before reviewing individual patients.
- Have individual informal meetings with members of the team to give them feedback and assess their own progress. These should be in addition to more formal forms of assessment.
- Give career advice when asked by juniors and show an interest in their career development. This can be a great cause of anxiety both for doctors unsure as to which specialty to pursue and those unsure of how to break into a training programme.
- Brief discussions at the start of each week will allow you, as head of the team, to know what is happening to all team members – who is on nights, who is on annual leave, which clinics are being covered by whom, and so on.

- The setting of goals should be both team-based and individual. Examples might be improving discharge summaries to GPs by all members of the team, or ensuring that one of the junior doctors passes a particular exam by the time she leaves the team.
- Social events should be regular and inclusive. For example, if you have a member of the team who doesn't drink alcohol, or one with family commitments who needs to leave early, then buying the whole team coffee and having a break before the end of the day may be a way to be inclusive.

Hospital management structure

Management in NHS hospitals in the UK varies between Trusts, but there are many similarities. It is worth knowing what the structure is in your own Trust, and this information will be readily available on the Trust's website. The exact roles may have different names and the interactions between people in the Trust will be slightly different, but broadly speaking the main players in the hospital's management structure are as described here.

- *Chief executive*. This is the most senior manager who is effectively the boss of the hospital. The CE may have a business background in addition to NHS experience. The CE has a number of roles, encompassing business performance of the Trust, financial results, maintaining the hospital's organisational structure and providing strategic direction. He or she reports directly to the chairman and the board of directors.
- *Chairman*. The chairman's role is usually to lead the board of directors. He or she shares overall leadership of the hospital Trust with the chief executive. The chairman leads all board meetings and is responsible for the running of meetings and the tasks arising from meetings.
- *Board of governors*. These are senior members who do not directly work in the hospital. They may work elsewhere or may be retired from the NHS or from the world of business. They will meet on a regular basis (perhaps monthly or quarterly) and provide a voice for the strategic direction of the Trust and for forming a long-term plan. They will also be responsible for appointing key personnel such as the chief executive.
- *Directors*. Directors are senior managers who usually report to the chief executive. Non-executive directors work for the Trust part-time. They often have another main job in the business sector and may sit on multiple boards, giving their advice and expertise at board meetings.

However, full-time hospital directors have busy full-time jobs in running the hospital. They will have specific roles in the hospital set-up, including directors of finance, operations, estates, nursing, clinical governance, human resources, and Trust performance.

- *Divisions*. These are divisions within the hospital which each has its own clinical and management structure. Typical examples are divisions of medicine, surgery, pathology, psychiatry, and paediatrics.

Self management

Managing your own time

In addition to managing your team, there will be increasing demands on your own time as you become a more senior doctor. There will be increased responsibility for patients (perhaps associated with a reduction in direct bedside care), requests for teaching medical students, someone asking you to help with an audit, increasing paperwork, training committee requests, and so on. It is important that you are able to manage your time wisely to make the most of any opportunities that you wish to pursue.

- Remember that your primary focus as a clinical doctor is patient care and this should take priority over all else.
- Try to stratify your tasks into those of high and low priority and shift your focus to deadlines with high priority.
- Put effort into areas that will further your own chosen area of interest. For example, teaching students and completing formal teaching qualifications may be more helpful than assisting with clinical research if medical education is where your passion lies.
- Keep an electronic list of tasks. It is all to easy to get swamped with emails and updates, but keeping a simple online task list that you can access from a smartphone or computer can be a way to keep on top of things to do.
- Always know when to say no, especially if the ask of you is too difficult or will consume too much time.
- Set yourself realistic deadlines and ensure that you keep to these as much as possible. Unrealistic timelines can be a source of considerable stress.
- Only multitask if you are able to do so efficiently. Research has shown that people who concentrate on specific tasks are often able to complete more in the same period of time than those who multitask.

- Give yourself rewards to look forward to. It might be something as simple as a glass of wine after a busy on call, or something more extravagant such as buying yourself a new car once you pass your final exams.
- As with all tasks in your career, the old adage of 'underpromise but overdeliver' is worth sticking too.

Managing stress

Stress in a doctor can be acute or chronic. It can range from the sudden stress as a medical doctor on call when faced with a cardiac arrest scenario, or the more gradual onset of stress experienced by a GP with paperwork building up and surgery finances to manage. A small amount of stress is good for a productive working atmosphere, but there is a fine line between productive work and being unable to work.

- Try to identify particular stress triggers and devise ways to avoid them or reduce the level of stress in that situation. For example, doing an outpatient clinic with a particular consultant may cause stress and anxiety, so aim to prepare for this where possible.
- Use simple stress-relieving techniques as appropriate. Good examples are getting enough sleep, avoidance of large quantities of alcohol, healthy eating, and regular exercise.
- Seek help to limit your stress when needed. Make sure you have a GP and visit him/her for advice, or speak to senior colleagues about their own methods for relieving stress.
- Make time for yourself daily. You might go to a gym, spend quality time with your partner or play computer games – whatever you need to relax, make sure you do it every day.
- Avoid burning out. Taking regular holidays, perhaps going away with family or friends in your annual leave rather than staying at home.
- Regularly rethink and edit your to-do list. If you find that it has grown too big then simply remove tasks that provide very little benefit.
- Accept that some things, whether at work or in your career progression, are simply out of your control (e.g. the paucity of consultant posts in your specialty). Learn to accept this as a way of dealing with stress rather than dwelling on it.

Managing your life outside medicine

In addition to managing your work it is vital that you are able to keep up to date with whatever else life throws at you. There is no point being a fantastic doctor if you are late with your mortgage payments, bad at relationships, keep putting off going home to see your parents, or are simply too busy to get a haircut. As with the rules for managing your work, similar tips can help with managing your home life and your work–life balance. Try to ensure that you are able to achieve progression in your desired career without sacrificing your own personal needs and ambitions.

Sources of further information

Global business practice: www.best-management-practice.com

GMC management for doctors: www.gmc-uk.org/guidance/ethical_guidance/management_for_doctors.asp

Google tasks: mail.google.com/mail/help/tasks/

Time management: www.selfgrowth.com/timemgt.html

11

Fellowships and working abroad

Key aims of this chapter

- Discuss the reasons for undertaking a fellowship or working abroad
- Give advice on applying for positions
- Suggest how to fund your time abroad.

Introduction

Whether to quench a desire to travel, experience other healthcare systems or gain specific clinical experience, spending time abroad or 'out of programme' (OOP) is popular. It is also regarded by most deaneries as a worthwhile experience.

Part of making the decision involves establishing what you want to accomplish by time spent abroad or out of programme. Is it a defined set of skills (e.g. trauma experience, endovascular training, exposure to HIV medicine), personal development (e.g. train for the Olympics), research, something different, or simply that you need 'time out'? Your answer will determine not only where you go and what you do, but also the timing and length of your new experience. This will need to be decided well ahead of your departure date, typically a year in advance.

Making sense of OOPCs, OOPEs and OOPTs

How do I seek approval?

If you are in a recognised training post, to take time 'out of programme' you will need to seek and gain approval from your postgraduate dean or deputy. This is usually achieved by first seeking approval from your training programme director (TPD) or chair of the STC (Specialty Training Committee) or heads of school.

Discussions relating to any OOP should occur almost as soon as the idea is conceived. Not only will this gauge the feasibility of the proposal before you start doing the legwork, but you may also get some useful advice or assistance in securing a fellowship or the position you want. Also, taking an OOP is likely to have human resource implications which can be more easily ironed out earlier than later. Your TPD will usually handle any negotiations on this front, but if your absence is likely to cause disruption you should also keep the necessary representatives of the Trust informed (Box 11.1).

The 'Gold Guide' (*A Reference Guide for Postgraduate Specialty Training in the UK*, published by the Department of Health) is an extremely useful document. It gives an overview of the national guidelines for allowing trainees to take time out of their specialty training programme. However, each deanery may have variations in terms of policy and requirements; so, rather than make assumptions, you should contact your deanery for advice. In general, no more than three years of specialty training may be taken OOP, but in reality this time can be flexible.

- If you are NOT in a training programme, make note of when applications for the next round of posts commence before you go away. Moreover, ensure you're in a position to both apply for and attend any interviews and not stranded in the middle of nowhere at these times.
- Maintain an up-to-date CV and logbook. Even if a post does not count towards training it is useful to maintain your portfolio with the necessary number or work-based assessments etc., as evidence of ongoing personal development.
- Maintain contact with your deanery and make sure you give sufficient notice of your intention to return to the programme. Not only will this ensure that the deanery and your programme director can slot you back into a post on your return, the post is more likely to be relevant to your needs.

Box 11.1 Tips for your time abroad

Types of OOP activity

Approved clinical training – OOPT (out of programme training)

Time taken out on an OOPT counts towards your certificate of completion of training (CCT), so your date for achieving your CCT will not alter. These posts require prospective approval by the General Medical Council with an application submitted to them directly from the deanery concerned. Notably, the GMC does not accept applications directly from trainees or the respective royal colleges.

To apply for an OOPT you need to complete the necessary application forms available from your deanery website, at least 6 months ahead of your proposed departure. For medicine trainees, a Joint Royal Colleges of Physicians Training Board (JRCPTB) form also needs to be completed and submitted to the deanery. Once the OOPT is approved by the deanery, they will then approach the GMC for approval of the post for training.

Importantly, while on your OOPT you will also be asked to continue to submit assessments (e.g. work-based) as if you were training in the UK, as well as undertake an annual review of competence progression (ARCP) or an equivalent process. This achieves a number of goals: it renews your commitment and registration to the training programme, requests permission to retain your national training number (NTN), and provides information about your likely date of return to the programme and date that you will complete training.

Other OOP types

Time may be taken out for reasons that may not count for training, and these therefore do not require prospective GMC approval. These periods away will result in a commensurate delay in the award of your CCT and can fall into one of the following categories:

- *Experience* – OOPE. This is a period that, although benefiting you in terms of exposure to different healthcare systems/environments or diseases, does not have a formal curriculum for training and thus is not considered as a training post. An example is a year abroad working for a charitable health agency, such as Médecins Sans Frontières (MSF) or Voluntary Services Overseas (VSO).
- *Research* – OOPR. This may be to undertake an MD or PhD. Part of this period in research can be counted towards your CCT if, for example, you also have some clinical commitments. However, you will need to apply for approval by the GMC prospectively.

● *Career break* – OOPC. This could be a planned career break from the specialty training, for example, to play rugby for New Zealand.

Fellowships

Be very clear why you want to embark on an out-of-programme experience. It may be that you are between posts having failed to secure a core training position (in which case your time away is not strictly classified as an OOP), or that you want to experience training abroad. If the latter, are you best placed to gain these skills in the middle of your training, in your final years of training, or post-CCT (i.e. a post-CCT fellowship)? Are there any prerequisites you will need to fulfill? For example, to work in the USA you need to have completed your American licensing examinations – the USMLEs (see Chapter 3). Also, is the post you're looking at suitable for you? For example, a fellowship in endovascular surgery is usually undertaken towards the end of training and the expectation is that applicants are senior trainees; you therefore won't get a look in if you apply to these positions as a year 1 specialist trainee.

How do I find opportunities?

Like most things in medicine, finding a suitable fellowship takes perseverance as well as luck. You probably have an idea of what you want to do, so you need to have the conviction that you can carry it through. If you have setbacks the key is to keep searching, however demoralised you feel.

Most fellowship posts will be advertised, but be aware that by the time that happens there will be other applicants who have already started the groundwork for that post. This groundwork can take a number of forms, including asking their boss to make email contact enquiring about the post, making contact with the head of department themself, either by email or at a meeting, or visiting the department either informally or as part of an organised observership (Box 11.2). The old adage, 'If you don't ask, you don't get' very much holds true, and most departments would rather take on someone who has taken the initiative and made the effort beforehand, or who they have some knowledge of or have been introduced to, rather than a complete stranger.

Where do I start?

● Email the heads of all departments in the area you would like to work, with a copy of your CV. Explain why you would like to work for them and enquire if there are any opportunities. This can be a tedious

Observerships are approved attachments to a department. They can range in length from a few days to a few months. As the title suggests, these positions enable you to watch procedures, patient histories, and physical examinations. Observers are usually also permitted to take part in other workings of a department (e.g. to attend patient ward rounds and teaching conferences), as well as utilise medical facilities, such as the library.

Most hospitals will have an International Medical Department, who you can get in touch with to organise these attachments. However, it is useful to contact first the physician you would like to shadow, to ascertain whether it is feasible for you to visit.

Importantly, observerships do not attract a salary and do not count as training.

Box 11.2 Observerships

process, and don't be disheartened if you do not get any replies at all from the dozens of departments you contact. Be persistent (without venturing into harassment).
- Introduce yourself to a potential boss at a meeting and ask about opportunities, or express an interest in visiting informally.
- Organise an informal visit to the department, or an observership. Observerships (see Box 11.2) are short approved attachments to a department, which can range in length from a few days to a few months.
- Look for advertisements for posts in the *British Medical Journal*, on Doctors.net and on deanery and specialist trainee group websites. The latter exist mainly for the surgical specialties – examples are the Rouleaux Club for vascular surgery and the Dukes Club for colorectal Surgery (Table 11.1).
- Speak to trainees who are currently in-post or who have done the post previously, not only about the job but also how to apply and who to speak to. Often a recommendation from them can go a long way in helping you to secure a job.

Seeing to the paperwork

Once you have secured the job of your dreams, if it is abroad, there is more work to do and you should not underestimate how time-consuming the paperwork can be to complete. You should be allocated a case worker

Table 11.1: Summary of subspecialty trainee groups

Specialty association	Specialty	Website
Association of Surgeons in Training (ASiT)	All surgeons in training	www.asit.org
Association of Surgeons of Great Britain and Ireland (ASGBI)	All surgical specialties	www.asgbi.org.uk
Rouleaux Club	Vascular surgery	rouleauxclub.com
Dukes Club	Colorectal surgery	www.thedukesclub.org.uk
Carrel Club	Transplant surgery	www.carrelclub.org.uk
British Orthopaedic Trainees Association (BOTA)	Orthopaedic surgery	www.bota.org.uk
Senior Urological Registrars Group (SURG)	Urology	www.surg-online.net
Academy's Trainee Doctors' Group (ATDG), Royal College of Physicians	Medicine	www.aomrc.org.uk/atdg-members.html
The Mammary Fold	Breast surgery	www.themammaryfold.com
Society of Academic and Research Surgery (SARS)	Generic surgical academic society	surgicalresearch.org.uk
Association of Otolaryngologists in Training (AOT)	Otolaryngology	www.aotent.com
Oromaxillofacial Trainees Group	Maxillofacial surgery	www.baoms.org.uk
British Neurosurgical Trainees Association	Neurosurgery	www.sbns.org
Paediatric Surgery Trainees Group	Paediatric surgery	groups.yahoo.com/group/paediatricsurgerytrainees
Surgical Oncology Trainee Association (SOTA)	Surgical oncology	www.baso.org/sota.aspx
Association of Cancer Surgery	Cancer surgery	www.baso.org
Association of Upper Gastrointestinal Surgeons (AUGIS) Trainees Group	Upper GI surgery	www.augis.org

who will guide you through the process, but the following will need to be organised.

Registration with the appropriate medical body

This can take anywhere between four and eight weeks. As part of the process you may be required to get verification of your basic medical degree from the Electronic International Credentials Service (EICS) of the Educational Commission for Foreign Medical Graduates of the United States (ECFMG), which will delay the processing of your application. Other documents required may include:

- proof of identity, such as certified copies of the biopage of your passport and driving licence
- your CV
- a letter from your secondary school stating you were a student at the school, your attendance dates at the school, and that your schooling was undertaken in English (certified copy or original)
- a letter of appointment to your position
- position description and training plan (this is usually provided by your employing body)
- certified copies of your medical and other degrees
- an original certified copy of a certificate of internship or letter from a medical registration authority confirming your completion of internship or other relevant documentation that establishes internship completion (this can be obtained from your medical school registry or foundation school)
- certificate of good standing (obtained by contacting the General Medical Council).

Visa and/or work permit

You will need to obtain a work visa, and often the organisation who will be employing you will sponsor your application. Depending on the country, visa requirements vary from sending certified copies of your passport biopage, and demonstrating evidence that you have health insurance in place to having a medical, chest x-ray and blood tests. Many countries operate an online visa application service, which makes the whole process a lot smoother than it would otherwise be.

Other documents

Obtaining your registration with the relevant medical board/council and your work visa are perhaps the most stressful parts of the application process. Once these are in place you can relax somewhat. Other factors you should also consider are:

- Do I have the necessary vaccinations?
- Do I need a foreign currency account for the country I will work in?
- What about health insurance? This may be covered by your travel insurance for short periods abroad, but for longer periods you might need to sign up to a healthcare plan. Many are available specifically designed for sabbaticals. You should also investigate whether you will be working in a country that has reciprocal health arrangements with the UK. If that's the case, you will not require additional health cover.
- Do I need medical malpractice insurance?
- What about accommodation? This may be provided, but more likely you will need to rent a home. Although it is tempting to find an apartment before you arrive, if you are new to an area and unfamiliar with it, you should book into a long-stay hotel initially. This should not stop you looking beforehand, and there are usually agents in the locality that will cater to sabbaticals or short-term lets. If you know people in the area, or even the person you are replacing in the post, they will be able to point you in the right direction – or even better, you might be able to take over their residence once they've left!

Other fellowships or experiences to consider

In addition to fellowships that enhance your clinical experience, periods of time spent in management, education and in developing leadership skills are gaining in popularity and are viewed in high regard. Below is a selection of opportunities in the aforementioned fields which are well worth considering.

The Harkness Fellows in Health Care Policy and Practice

Previously known as the Commonwealth Fund Fellowships, the Harkness Fellowships are run by the Commonwealth Fund of New York City (NYC). They offer participants the opportunity to gain insight and an appreciation of the US healthcare system, with the option to develop their research skills and develop contacts and forge collaborative work. The fellowship is for a one-year period and is undertaken at an American institution such as Harvard University, Columbia University, Stanford University, or Johns Hopkins University.

Fellowships in clinical leadership

Previously known as Darzi Fellowships, these are run by NHS London's Leading for Health and the London Deanery in collaboration with the King's Fund. They are full-time 12-month programmes allowing GPs in training, newly qualified GPs and specialist registrars to develop leadership skills in acute, foundation, mental health and primary care settings. Participants are typically mentored by their medical director and over the year given the opportunity to lead on a variety of projects within their Trusts, on areas such as service change, quality/safety improvement and leadership skills development.

Fellowships in medical education

Aimed at specialty registrars, these positions allow participants to gain experience and develop their skills as medical educators. An FME lasts 6 months, and fellows are attached to an 'education unit' within a London NHS Trust. Posts run from February to April or from August to October. FME posts at the time of writing were available at the following: St Barts and the London NHS Trust; Imperial College Healthcare NHS Trust; North Middlesex University Hospital Trust; North West London Hospitals Trust; and Tavistock and Portman NHS Foundation Trust.

Charitable organisations

The options to work abroad in a charitable capacity are endless, but they can take time to organise. Volunteering for a medical charity or an aid and development organisation offers you the opportunity to travel and work in different countries and experience different healthcare systems, often under very challenging but equally very rewarding conditions. In addition, if it is in a field you are interested in pursuing, then it can provide suitable skills and contacts to make a break into that field.

Although there are programmes available that will charge you to participate, many organisations exist that can provide for your basic needs (accommodation, food etc.) in exchange for your medical expertise. The well-established organisations will also take care of the necessary paperwork, which can be like wading through treacle in some countries and impossible to achieve as an individual in others. Examples of charitable medical organisations are given below.

Médecins Sans Frontières

MSF is a politically neutral and impartial private international medical humanitarian organisation created by doctors and journalists in France in 1971. Its aim is to provide assistance to populations in distress, victims of natural or man-made disasters, and victims of armed conflict – irrespective of race, religion, creed or political convictions. MSF is made up mainly of doctors and health sector workers who work in nearly 60 countries. There is no age limit. However, volunteers are expected to have at least two years' professional experience in their area of specialisation.

The average mission period is 6 months. Volunteers undertake missions on the understanding that, regardless of how dangerous the mission is, they will not make a claim for themselves or their assigns for any form of compensation other than what the association might be able to afford them. Their website is www.msf.org.uk.

Walking with Maasai

This is a non-profit organisation established by and for the Maasai communities in the Olorte region of southern Kenya. As part of its aim to build a stronger Maasai future, it is involved in developing healthcare initiatives that reduce the burden of preventable disease, and running education programmes that enable the Maasai to improve the effectiveness and sustainability of their use of the land. A small, little-known charity, it has the potential to offer great experience of working in remote areas. However, expenses are likely to be borne by you. Their website is www.walkingwithmaasai.org.

Remote Area Medical Volunteer Corps

This is a non-profit, volunteer, airborne relief corps which provides free healthcare, dental care, eye care and technical and educational assistance to people in remote areas of the USA and the world. Volunteers participate in expeditions at their own expense. The website is www.ramusa.org.

Doctors of the World UK

This is part of the Médecins du Monde network, an international aid organisation that provides medical care and empowers vulnerable people such as victims of natural disasters, famine and diseases (endemic or epidemic, particularly AIDS), victims of armed conflicts and political violence, refugees, displaced people, minority populations, street children, drug users, and all people with no access to healthcare. It operates in over 70 countries worldwide and missions typically last between 6 and 12 months. Their website is www.medecinsdumonde.org.uk.

Flying Doctors of America

They provide medical assistance to as many of the poor and needy they are able to reach by flying medical and dental teams to areas in need. The website is www.fdoamerica.org.

Mercy Ships

This provides free surgery and medical care, and works with local communities to improve healthcare. Volunteers are expected to raise their own finances to become crew members, paying towards the cost of living on board, insurance, and transportation to and from the service location. Placements range from two weeks to one year. Long-term crews make an initial commitment of two years. The website is www.mercyships.org.uk.

Health Volunteers Overseas

HVO is a network of healthcare professionals, organisations, corporations and donors united in the common aim to improve global health through education. It achieves this by sending qualified professionals overseas to train local healthcare providers and currently has clinical education training programmes running in more than 25 countries. HVO also runs a number of fellowship programmes, including the Young Surgeon Traveling Fellowship, Orthopaedics Traveling Fellowships, and the Society for Education in Anesthesia (SEA) Traveling Fellowship. The website is www.hvousa.org.

Funding arrangements

The majority of OOPs are funded and there is an associated salary. However, this may not hold true for all posts, such as observerships, OOPRs and OOPEs. What you plan to do in your out-of-programme period will dictate the potential funding streams you can tap into. Funding can be obtained from a number of sources, including:

- your specialty college (Royal College of Surgeons, Royal College of Physicians etc.)
- specialty organisations and charities (e.g. Circulation Foundation)
- local medical charities (e.g. the Simpson–Smith Travelling Prize)
- charitable organisations (e.g. Wellcome Trust, Royal Society of Medicine)

Table 11.2: Examples of sources of funding

	Awarding organisation	Amount	Frequency	Applicants	Purpose
Research					
Norman Capener Travelling Fellowship	RCS(Eng)	Variable	Biennial	Higher surgical trainees, with interest in orthopaedic or hand surgery	To pursue a research project that involves travelling
HJ Windsor Prize	RCS(Eng), from Ethicon Foundation Fund	£500	NA	An Australian or British surgeon	To pursue a research or educational project in Australia or British Isles
Sir Ratanji Dalal Research Scholarship	RCS(Eng)	£20 000	Annual	All medical practitioners	To support a project in tropical medicine or surgery
Daniel Turnberg UK/ Middle East Travel Fellowship	RCS(Eng)	£3500	NA	Clinical and non-clinical researchers	Opportunity to undertake short-term visits to learn techniques or develop experience in countries in the Middle East
Norman Gamble Grant	Royal Society of Medicine	£1500	Annual	Lay and medical applicants	Research in otology
Clinical experience					
Ethicon Foundation Fund	RCS(Eng)	£400	NA	Fellow or member of the college	Travel to UK or Europe to further enhance specialty skill or experience
Colledge Family Memorial Fellowship Fund	RCS(Eng)	£10 000	Annual	Senior trainee or new consultant in otolaryngology or head and neck surgery	A study (clinical or research) period overseas

Award	Organisation	Amount	Frequency	Eligibility	Purpose
Ronald Raven Barbers Award	RCS(Eng)	£1500	Biennial	Trainee surgeons in the UK	Assist in learning a new surgical technique or procedure
Ellison–Cliffe Travelling Fellowship	Royal Society of Medicine	£15 000	Annual	Fellows of the RSM of specialist registrar or lecturer grade, or within 3 years of consultant appointment	Cover expenses to travel abroad to 1–2 centres for >6 months for study, research or clinical training
Neil Med Travelling Fellowship	Royal Society of Medicine	£1000	Annual	UK registrars and senior registrars in otolaryngology and consultants within one year of appointment who are Fellows of the RSM	Travel to a rhinology or head and neck unit
Ophthalmology Section Travelling Fellowship	Royal Society of Medicine	£1000	Biennial	British-based ophthalmologists travelling abroad and foreign ophthalmologists travelling to the UK	Study or advancement of ophthalmology
Otology Section Training Scholarship	Royal Society of Medicine	£1000	Annual	Trainee in otology	Visit a centre to gain experience in otology
Venous Forum Travelling Fellowship	Royal Society of Medicine	£1000	Annual	Surgical trainees with an interest in venous disease	Travel to a centre to gain expertise in venous disease
Moynihan Travelling Fellowship	Association of Surgeons of Great Britain and Ireland	£5000	Annual	Specialist registrars towards the end of specialty training	To broaden their education

(Continued)

Table 11.2: *(Continued)*

	Awarding organisation	Amount	Frequency	Applicants	Purpose
Dame Sheila Sherlock Travelling Fellowship	Royal College of Physicians	£2000	Annual	Consultants and trainees	Opportunity to learn new techniques and acquire new experiences, ideas and stimulation through travel; for 1-month periods
Samuel Leonard Simpson Fellowships in Endocrinology	Royal College of Physicians	£8000	Annual	Those suitably qualified	To learn new techniques and acquire new experiences, ideas and stimulation through travel and the exchange of ideas in endocrinology
John Glyn Bursary in Rheumatology	Royal College of Physicians	NA	Annual	UK consultants and specialist registrars	To support travel and other costs associated with a visit to another centre in the UK or abroad, for the purpose of learning new clinical or research techniques relevant to rheumatology

- travelling prizes associated with meetings (e.g. Venous Forum Travelling Fellowship)
- pharmaceutical companies.

The list of potential donors is extensive. With regard to the last-named, in the current economic climate this can be a difficult route to pursue. It might be useful if you or your consultant have, over time, built a rapport with a particular company. Otherwise it literally is a case of cold-calling.

Table 11.2 has a selection of the prizes available. Although competition for these funds is often fierce, that is not a reason not to apply.

Sources of further information

Harkness fellowships: www.commonwealthfund.org/Fellowships/Harkness-Fellowships.aspx

Joint Royal Colleges of Physicians Training Board: www.jrcptb.org.uk

NHS clinical leadership: www.nhsleadership.org/workstreams-clinical-fellowshipprogramme.asp

12

Becoming a specialist: the rabbit in the hat

Key aims of this chapter

- How to make the most of your training years and plan the next phase of your career
- The hospital consultant person specification
- Alternatives to a standard medical career.

Introduction

Even for all those who have done research, completed audits, gone on teaching courses and management away days, it can still be very difficult to stand out from the crowd. The job market is tough, and never has competition been fiercer, with candidate-to-post ratios being reported as high as 100 to 1 in some specialties for hospital consultant posts. For all of these reasons you need to try to stand out from your peers as you move through specialist training. This chapter consolidates much of what has been discussed throughout this book and in the earlier companion book (*Royal Society of Medicine Career Handbook: FY1 – ST2*). However, sometimes you need to do something radically different and – like all good magicians – you need to pull a rabbit out of a hat.

Planning your career

It is difficult to see how things will ease up in the near future; but, as a young trainee, rather than give up and throw away years of hard work and a career that gives you a high level of job satisfaction, the best you can do is make sure you're the best person for the job when it does come up.

This, however, does not happen overnight. It takes years of careful consideration and planning. Moreover, your perspective on what is the perfect job for you is likely to change over your specialty training, undoubtedly being influenced by personal circumstances and other external factors. It is therefore important to keep evaluating your position and not be afraid of seeking help or advice if you are at a crossroads or are having second thoughts about your chosen career pathway. Remember, no one job suits all. While an academic or full-time clinical career is for some, a more flexible or family-friendly post may be for you.

As you become more senior it is useful to have a roadmap of where you wish to go. This could be in your head, drawn on the back of a beer mat, or made professionally as a chart using the latest software. The map should display your key obstacles (e.g. exams, job competition) and your own clinical specialist deficiencies. It can also detail ways to tackle these hurdles – for example, applying for a specialist fellowship overseas to learn a particular new skill that may be invaluable when you come back home and apply for jobs. The roadmap can constantly change as you change your own outlook on the ideal career pathway.

In some respects, your years as a specialty registrar are the hardest of your career and there will be both highs and lows. There will be the excitement of having a greater degree of independence and constantly learning new skills, and this will be coupled with greater responsibility not only to your patients but also to more junior members of the team. This may be compounded by the stress of a long commute (which can be miserable especially in the winter months), studying for postgraduate exams or writing up a thesis, and the pressure to be constantly producing publications in your spare time along with juggling a home life. It is not an uncommon finding for trainees to report that it is difficult to 'let go' at the end of the day, but it is important that you do develop a life outside medicine – be it spending quality time with your family or a close group of friends. It is vital that you have an established outlet to vent your stresses.

Making the most of your specialty years

The easiest place to start is to take a look at what the expectations are for applicants to a consultant post, and it is never too early to do this. Although you might feel a little overwhelmed initially, if you take a closer look, the skills and characteristics expected of you are very achievable over the five or six years of specialty training – and indeed, many build upon skills you will have already acquired. Moreover, it is far better to be prepared too early, then to reach your final year of training and realise that there are key gaps in your CV that could very easily have been plugged with some prior consideration.

Consultant jobs: the person specification

The person specification for a post outlines the necessary requirements in terms of training, clinical experience and personal characteristics you need in order to apply. You will be expected to demonstrate aspects of the person specification in your consultant application form, CV and finally, when you are shortlisted, in the interview. The person specification usually describes some criteria as being non-negotiable (e.g. registration on the specialty register), and others as being desirable. Although the latter are not mandatory, given the competitiveness of the jobs market, you will be at a clear advantage over other candidates and are more likely to be shortlisted if you possess as many of them as possible. That said, you need only be as good as the competition, and even if you do not fulfil some areas of the criteria, you may more than make up for this in other areas.

The person specification is typically divided into eight broad categories (outlined in Box 12.1) and these are based on the General Medical Council's document *Good Medical Practice*.

- Basic qualifications and higher degrees
- Special interests and fellowships
- Clinical governance:
  - audit
  - research
  - management
  - teaching
- Personal attributes

Box 12.1 Overview of the person specification

Qualifications

As a specialty trainee you will have the necessary recognised medical qualifications. Overseas trainees may in addition to their basic qualification have undertaken the Professional and Linguistics Assessments Board (PLAB) exam. In addition to these, there are a number of courses and degrees that you could undertake to improve your prospects.

Hospital doctors will need to have taken higher (exit or subspecialty) postgraduate examinations in order to apply for consultant posts. For example, as a surgical trainee you will require the FRCS examination in your subspecialty, and for the medical specialties the appropriate exit qualification if applicable (see Chapter 3). Additionally, in order to be eligible to apply for a consultant post you will need either to be on the GMC's specialist register or be within six months of completion of your certificate of completion of training (CCT).

Special interests and fellowships

Apart from being able to show a breadth of experience by the posts you have undertaken and your logbook, you will need to demonstrate an interest in your subspecialty. This will in part be reflected by your subspecialty choice in your exit exam (if applicable), but your last 1–2 years of specialty training should also be in your subspecialty area. For example, if you are a renal medicine trainee and have an interest in hypertension management, years 5 and/or 6 of training could be spent in a tertiary specialist unit. You could also develop a research interest and have publications in this field, which would further demonstrate your interest in this area.

Although specialisation and subspecialisation are being advocated at an earlier stage, be wary about declaring a subspecialty interest too early, especially in a niche area, as this will limit the posts you can apply for. For example, a cardiologist might in some units be expected to participate in the general medical on-call rota, and in other units be on a separate cardiology-only rota. So, if at the end of training you are not comfortable with general medical on-calls, you would be limited to applying to the latter posts. This, however, might be a deliberate career choice on your part.

In some specialties you may need to gain competency in a specific technique in order to prove attractive to a future employee; examples are endoscopy and laparoscopic skills for upper and lower GI surgeons, endovascular skills for vascular surgery, and so on. An overseas or national fellowship is a well-recognised method of achieving these specialty-specific skills (see Chapter 11) and is well worth considering in the later years of training. These fellowships can be taken as an out-of-programme (OOP) experience and may be counted towards training (OOPT). They do, however, require forward thinking and planning, and prior permission needs to be obtained from your deanery.

Experience at consultant grade or demonstration of the ability to take full and independent responsibility for the clinical care of patients will be an advantage; and when you are ready, you should seize the opportunity to act-up if it arises. It may be that you are asked to cover a sick colleague, or you may be recommended for a locum position. A locum post is a good foot in the door to consultancy as there is a high likelihood of a locum position being advertised in the future as a more permanent post. Moreover, as somebody in-house you have a high probability of getting the job, provided you play your cards right (and if, of course, the Trust can afford to take you on).

Clinical governance

Courses and education

When applying for a consultant post you will be expected to demonstrate active participation in continuing medical education (CME) and continuing professional development (CPD). Although there is no formal requirement for this as a trainee, it is in some cases necessary and in other cases advisable, for you to undertake certain specialty-specific training courses, such as advanced trauma life support (ATLS) for surgeons and advanced life support (ALS) for physicians, as well as personal development courses (e.g. teaching and leadership skills courses). You have an annual study entitlement (typically 30 days) for this and allocated study leave funds (this will vary according to your deanery, and currently can range from £700 per annum in Oxford to £1950 per annum in South Yorkshire & South Humber). Both study leave and study funding need to be applied for prospectively – typically 4–6 weeks ahead of the proposed course. If you are having difficulty taking study leave, perhaps due to service commitments, you should speak initially to your supervising consultant or educational supervisor.

In addition to going on courses, attendance at key meetings in your specialty plays two key roles. It helps you to keep abreast of the important issues facing your specialty in terms of training and disease management, and it enables you to network and identify ahead of time any potential jobs that may arise.

Research or academic experience

It is unusual to be considered as a serious contender for a consultant post, especially in some of the more popular specialties or more popular regions, without having done some formal research, in the form of either an MD or PhD. Physicians usually undertake research during their specialty training, whereas surgical trainees more often embark on research between core and specialty training. There are also a number of academic posts that will facilitate ongoing research throughout your specialty training.

When applying for consultant posts, an understanding of research methodology, the ability to critically appraise scientific literature and to apply research outcomes to clinical problems is essential. Research prowess can be exemplified in a number of ways, including:

- participation in national clinical trials
- evidence of clinical research, resulting in publications (new clinical research should be commenced early, at the start of a job, as it can take time to obtain ethical approval for a study, recruit sufficient numbers of participants and motivate colleagues)
- evidence of supervision of junior colleagues to conduct clinical or non-clinical research
- publications in referenced journals (case reports, while useful as a foundation or core trainee, carry little weight at consultant level)
- presentation of clinical and non-clinical research at regional, national and international meetings (this not only gives an indicator of the calibre of your research, but also says that you have the ability to design and deliver talks effectively)
- prizes or awards related to research work.

Audit

You should have experience of audit from your foundation and core training years. However, owing to the brevity of foundation posts, you may not have yet had the opportunity to fully complete the audit loop, and more likely you would have either started the first part of an audit or been involved in the second part – completion of the audit cycle.

For consultant posts you need to be able to demonstrate not only experience of designing an audit programme (including seeking approval from your audit/clinical governance lead to perform the audit), but also completion of an audit in its entirety; and ideally the audit should be in an area pertinent to your specialty of choice. This doesn't, however, mean that you cannot enlist the help of your keen foundation or core trainees, who will also benefit from the experience. Where possible you should also participate in national audits or be aware of national audits in relation to your specialty. Discussion of any audits performed will prove useful at interview.

Leadership

Effective leadership can help an organisation to become more efficient, allowing it to maximise its potential and function to deliver a high-quality service to its stakeholders. It is, too, a key quality that employers look for when recruiting consultants. Leadership development is the process of identifying, building or nurturing the quality of leadership within an organisation, and the clinical leadership competency framework (CLCF) describes the leadership and management competences clinicians need in order to be involved in the planning, delivery and transformation of healthcare services within the NHS.

There are a number of initiatives that can help you as a trainee to develop your leadership skills. A handful of these are listed below:

● The 'clinical leadership programme' developed by BMJ Learning, in collaboration with the Open University Business School's Centre for Professional Learning and Development, sets out to 'equip clinical leaders with the right resources to develop their leadership talent and help them overcome barriers to realise their potential'. This is achieved through a series of online, work-based courses and qualifications in clinical leadership. Being an online resource, it has the advantage that it can be completed at your own pace, but it is expensive. The website is www.clp.bmj.com.

● The NHS Clinical Leaders Network (CLN) is a national, professional leadership network for clinicians in England. It acts to bring together 'local clinical champions to initiate positive, transformational change and spread good practice across the NHS, and aims to support clinical leadership and engagement, improve NHS clinical service delivery and enable clinicians to influence policy implementation by giving them direct access to local and national policy leads'. The website is www.cln.nhs.uk.

● The National Leadership Council (NLC) clinical leadership fellowships encourage and support fellows to lead 'on regional projects to improve quality standards and efficiency and enables them to develop their leadership capability whilst delivering business critical improvements'. The website is www.nhsleadership.org.

- The NHS Prepare to Lead scheme is London-based. It is undertaken on a part-time basis over one year. It aims to support clinicians who have the potential to become future healthcare leaders to progress more smoothly into GP and consultant posts that have significant Trust or strategic level management and leadership responsibilities. Participants are assigned a mentor, typically a senior healthcare leader, and spend time shadowing their mentor, working with him or her on small projects or attending events and networking opportunities. In addition, they attend seminars or workshops throughout the year. The website is www.london.nhs.uk/leading-for-health/programmes/prepare-to-lead.
- A three-day course on 'clinical management and leadership' at Keele University is directed specifically at specialist registrars (SpRs) in their final years of training. It aims to 'prepare SpRs for the transition from training to independent specialist practice at consultant level, focusing on the management tasks, issues and problems likely to be faced by today's consultants'. Each day is themed and linked in to the medical leadership competency framework (MLCF). The website is www.keele.ac.uk/cml.

Management

Consultants are increasingly being asked to take on more and more managerial roles. As a senior trainee (and to-be-appointed-consultant) within the NHS, some key skills worth honing are an understanding of NHS organisational, structural and functional processes. This includes an understanding of the following:

- your Trust's goals and performance objectives
- the aims and objectives of internal and external agencies
- clinical governance, risk management and adverse-incident reporting
- appraisal and revalidation.

Ultimately your Trust will be looking to employ a dynamic individual who will take responsibility for delivering quality patient care, who has a commitment to audit and clinical governance, and who will work with management to deliver on Trust goals and objectives. Your willingness to contribute may be demonstrated, for example, by your ability in the past to help organise services (e.g. waiting lists, outpatient services) so that they run more efficiently, or perhaps your proven ability to facilitate change by working hard to identify and overcome barriers. Alternatively, you may have a track record for being a trouble-shooter, so when presented with a plan you identify problems and are able to come up with suitable alternatives.

Finding management opportunities

- *Courses on management, leadership, appraisal and revalidation.* Although there are a number of courses out there that form a useful introduction to the topic (and part of the tick-boxing process), management is best learnt by doing or seeing. You will also be surprised at how much you use management in your day-to-day activities.
- *Opportunities at work.* The key is to keep your eyes peeled. While the thought of organising the foundation or core training rota may fill you with dread, it will also teach you a number of skills – in particular, good communication and people/time management. Other managerial roles as a trainee could include:
  - ○ helping to develop a business plans (e.g. for purchasing equipment)
  - ○ advising on the efficient and smooth running of a specialist service
  - ○ managing a surgical firm
  - ○ coordinating the multidisciplinary team meetings
  - ○ managing your research budget.
- *Working with management.* It may also be possible and useful to develop links or to shadow senior managers within your current Trust. This will need to be coordinated around your clinical duties, but could potentially give you a great insight into their roles and the NHS management hierarchy.

Teaching experience

By this stage you and every other specialty trainee will have cited teaching or supervision of medical students, foundation and core trainees under the teaching section of their CV. As you progress you may also supervise more junior specialty trainees. The teaching can be informal, ranging from giving medical students or junior doctors tutorials to assessing clinical skills and giving lectures on your specialty (see Chapter 9 for details).

By the time you are at the stage of applying for a consultant post you should have a broad range of teaching styles to your armoury, and a good understanding of methods of delivering education and learning assessment tools. The latter may be developed through:

- attending teaching courses, such as the 'Teach the Teachers' or 'Training the Trainers' courses
- undertaking a one-year full-time or 2/3-year part-time or long-distance learning MSc in medical education, surgical education or other similar formal degree or certified course

- helping to develop revision or teaching courses
- undertaking the 'training and assessment in practice' (TAIP) course.

TAIP is a one-day course aimed at programme directors and educational supervisors. It imparts an appreciation of the training and assessment system and guides you through the assessment of higher trainees, from needs analysis, setting up a learning agreement to workplace-based assessment methods. Moreover, you will not be eligible to work as a consultant trainer if you are not TAIP-qualified.

Personal attributes

There are a number of attributes which span all of the categories and repeatedly crop up as desirable or essential characteristics in a consultant person specification. Ability to work and manage a team, communicate well, professionalism and flexibility are all qualities outlined in the GMC's document *Good Medical Practice*, but are also qualities that a department will look for when taking on a prospective colleague. A sample of these personal attributes are listed in Box 12.2.

The role of the deanery

Although there are a number of resources available to you dealing with careers planning, and your educational supervisor and annual review of competence progression (Box 12.3) will guide you, you are ultimately responsible for both record keeping and ensuring you are on track to your final destination, wherever that may be.

Record keeping is paramount in medicine, never more so than while you are in training. Essentially, if there is no record of it, you haven't done it! So update your CV and portfolio at regular intervals. Documents you should keep safe include:

- evidence of prizes or awards
- certificates from:
  - examinations
  - attendance at courses or meetings
- copies of publications and articles written
- evidence of out-of-work activities, such as formal and informal teaching or courses organised
- your portfolio with your required workplace-based assessments (this may be held as an e-portfolio)
- a logbook of procedures performed.

- Communicaton skills
  - possesses a high level of verbal and written communication skills
  - is able to communicate well with other members of the team, patients and relatives
  - possesses the necessary information technology (IT) skills.

- Teamwork
  - is able to work well within a team
  - is flexible – willing to cover for colleagues
  - is able to motivate staff, and facilitate appropriate changes in clinical practice
  - is able to represent the team in all forums
  - is approachable
  - is able to manage conflict appropriately by negotiation or decision making.

- Professional qualities
  - is honest, has integrity, and an appreciation of ethical dilemmas
  - has a caring attitude towards patients
  - possesses empathy, understanding and patience
  - is able to make clear rational decisions, exercising independent judgement in a professional and competent manner.

- Organisational skills
  - possesses good time-management skills
  - is able to prioritise tasks.

- Versatility and flexibility
  - is willing to undertake additional professional responsibilities at local, regional or national levels
  - is able to adapt to changing roles or circumstances
  - is able to cope under pressure.

- Commitment to clinical governance
  - has an enquiring and critical approach to work
  - learns from and shares experience and knowledge
  - is aware of own personal development needs
  - will take on responsibility and lead by example
  - is able to undertake appraisals and set personal development plans.

Box 12.2 Sample of personal attributes for a consultant

Each year as a specialty trainee you will undergo an ARCP. This replaced the RITA (record of in-training assessment) that is still undertaken by Calman Trainees.

The ARCP is a formal review of how you are progressing in terms of both your clinical ability and personal development. It is assessed using the evidence you present to your ARCP panel, which will typically be composed of the training programme director (TPD), members of the relevant specialty training committee (STC), a college representative, a deanery representative, an academic representative, and an 'external' or a lay representative. The outcome of the ARCP will determine whether you are allowed to progress to the next level of training.

Depending on your deanery, following review of the evidence (typically your portfolio, clinical logbook, CV and a structured report from your supervisor amongst other documents) you will be invited to discuss your short-term and long-term plans with the panel. Outcome following your ARCP will guide your CCT date. Repeated failure to produce adequate documentation, or under-performance, may lead to your ultimately being required to relinquish your National Training Number.

Box 12.3 The annual review of competence progression (ARCP)

The rabbit in the hat

Ultimately it is you who mostly controls the path of your career. Luck plays a part, and there will be times when a decision will send you down one path rather than another (for either better or worse). The key is to be open-minded and flexible; if you don't get into your desired fellowship one year, it's worth waiting to apply for it the next year.

If you imagine that most consultant jobs or GP partnerships are jobs for life, when you take on a post it will be potentially for 30 years or more. In that case, you should choose your consultant post wisely. In the current job market, one strategy is to prolong your training years with a variety of building blocks to add to your portfolio before you apply for your desired senior job.

With the option of out-of-programme experiences (OOPEs), you can make your specialty training as diverse or single-tracked as you want. There are endless opportunities. You could take a training or non-training year abroad, or undertake an MD/PhD or even an MBA. In addition, there are other options, such as joining the Royal Navy or Army. During your medical career and even late into your specialty training you may find yourself reconsidering your original game plan.

If the opportunity arises to do something as unique as an MBA or train for the Olympics, then it is important that you seriously consider the ramifications of both deciding to do it or not pursuing the opportunity. The primary disadvantage is that you will be prolonging your training, but this may be a wise decision if you are aiming for a competitive speciality. Additionally, there will be a significant drop in salary. You may even end up not only sacrificing your salary but also paying course fees – upwards of £30 000. There will also be family and friends to consider as you make these decisions.

Having said that, the advantages of a unique opportunity may significantly outweigh the disadvantages. A short-term salary drop may, in the long term, lead to an increased financial gain. Paying to attend a fellowship overseas learning endoscopy may lead you to a consultant post with significant private practice in that area. The unexpected is also a good talking point in any interview, and it may be that if you have scored highly in all other areas, the rabbit in the hat is enough to push you over the finish line.

Seeking help

If you need careers advice, there are a number of avenues you could pursue. Your educational supervisor, deanery and specialty training committee (STC) chair are useful first points of contact. Some other contacts are listed at the end of this chapter.

Leaving medicine

Leaving medicine is not a decision that anyone makes lightly. Apart from the time and money invested in studying and training, you are effectively making a leap from a job with reasonable job security and job satisfaction into the unknown. There are, however, a number of other happy endings to your working career if not in medicine, and over time be aware that you have accrued a number of so-called 'transferable skills' that can be applied in other work settings: team building; time, people and resource management; and communication skills.

It might not be that medicine is not for you, but that your chosen specialty is not for you. Clarify this in your mind. For example, would you enjoy the greater flexibility that comes with a career in general practice rather than a career in cardiothoracic surgery?

If it is definitely a career change you are after, there are a number of options. In fact there are endless options, including the well-trodden and established path into the legal profession or the pharmaceutical industry and other health-related industries.

Or perhaps you'd prefer something completely different ... .

Sources of further information

Joint RCP training board: www.jrcptb.org.uk/Pages/homepage.aspx

Modernising Medical Careers: www.mmc.nhs.uk

NHS Careers: www.nhscareers.nhs.uk

NHS Medical Careers: www.medicalcareers.nhs.uk/career_planning.aspx

13

Choosing your final job ... and the consultant interview

Key aims of this chapter

- Describe the decisions associated with choosing a final job
- Discuss the advantages and disadvantages of different types of final job
- Give tips on preparing for the consultant interview.

Introduction

Whether your final job is as a hospital consultant, associate specialist or staff grade, or as a GP or a ship's doctor, you will need to make your choice wisely. Although the old adage of 'a job for life' is no longer true for all doctors, many who finish their specialist training will settle on a final senior job that lasts for the majority of their career. For these reasons it is important that you make your decision carefully.

Moreover, once you have found your ideal job, it is vital that you make yourself as prepared as possible for the interview (senior GP interview tips are discussed in Chapter 2).

Choosing your final job

Location, location, location

As with buying property, the most important thing for you may be the location of your final job. However, there might not be an option in specialties where the number of posts nationwide is limited. For example, if you are interested in an academic post in a very specialised area, there may be just one or two places in the country that have the facilties to support your interests. In such cases, the decision is not the location but rather whether or not to pursue a niche career that may only allow you to apply to a limited number of places – and this decision needs to be made early in specialist training, not at the final hurdle.

However, for the majority of hospital doctors and GPs, the location is what will drive them towards applying for a final job. There are three main factors that need to be taken into account when considering the location.

Your clinical practice

Ask yourself, what are your needs and aspirations for your final job in the context of any advertised post.

- Is the clinical case mix the right one for you?
- Is the setting the right one for you (e.g. teaching hospital versus rural hospital)?
- Does it fit your own expertise?
- What is the on-call commitment?
- What is the weekly timetable like?
- Is there potential to grow as a senior doctor in the role?
- How friendly or difficult will your colleagues be?
- What potential is there for private practice?
- What potential is there to increase your NHS salary?
- How much administration is involved with the role?
- How long have other senior doctors been in position?
- How highly regarded is the institution?

Your home

This factor is important as it may be the place where you spend the rest of your working and retired life.

- What are house prices like in the region?
- Is there potential to buy better property as you become even more senior, but still within a short distance of work?
- How far will you need to commute in order to live in an affordable home but one that is right for your status in life? Generally, hospital doctors will need to live within a 20-minute drive or 10-mile radius of work for any on-call duties – even if you rarely have to go in at night.

- What amenities does the area have?
- What is the general quality of life like in the region?
- How far is it to motorways and the local airport?

Your family

This final factor is primarily for those who have children and partners.

- What are the local schools like?
- What are your other childcare options like?
- How safe is the local area?
- What opportunities are there for children outside of school hours?
- How close is your own family if needed for support (e.g. your siblings or parents)?
- How far is the location of work from your partner's place of work? Can you both easily commute to work if you took the post? Or would your partner need to consider leaving their job?

The familiar versus the new

Many people will apply for a consultant job in areas where they have worked as a trainee. This may be in the same hospital or in the training region within which they worked. The advantage is that you will know your future colleagues and the layout of the hospital, as well as know the set-up of the job and how the department works – including the internal politics (and every department has them). If you have got on well with them in the past, it may be that you are asked back for an interview. Prior to this you should visit the institution and have more detailed discussions with the consultants about the job itself and also about your chances of success. It is likely, but not always the case, that you will have a stronger chance of getting the job compared with someone who has not worked in the region before, all other things being equal. This does not mean, however, that you should prepare any less or work less hard for the interview.

You might, of course, decide to opt for a completely new start in a new region. This could be due to the need for a change, or for personal reasons. For example, after training in a big city you might decide to move to a more rural job to suit the schooling needs of your children and/or for a better quality of life. These are difficult decisions but ones that must be taken after much thought and discussion with all those involved, including your family.

Details of the job

Most job adverts contain very little detail about the exact terms and conditions. However, there will often be online links to the full details. There are a number of things to consider when reviewing the accompanying documentation (factors associated with GP senior posts are discussed in Chapter 4).

The job description

This is the central document housing most of the information regarding the specifics of the job you are seeking. This will include information on working conditions, rotas and support staff. It will also typically have general information about the hospital Trust, the university (if appropriate), and the local environment (brief details of travel links, schools etc.).

The job plan

This section will detail the number of PAs (programmed activities). The 2003 consultant contract is based on a full-time work commitment of 10 programmed activities (PAs) per week, each having a timetabled value of four hours. These can be split up into DCC (direct clinical care) and SPAs (supporting professional activities). A typical model for hospital consultant posts is 7.5 DCCs and 2.5 SPAs. A part-time post will not necessarily be for 5 PAs, so it is important when taking on a flexible post that you know the number of PAs you will be working, as this will directly affect your NHS salary.

DCC sessions include emergency duties, operating sessions, ward rounds, outpatient activities, clinical diagnostic work and multidisciplinary meetings. SPAs include training, medical education, continuing professional development, formal teaching, audit, appraisal, research, management and clinical governance activities.

The weekly schedule

It is vital that you drill down into the specifics of the weekly timetable as you may be stuck with it for the rest of your life! Find out how often the on-calls are worked, whether they are resident on-call and, if not, how often it is likely that you will be asked to come in. There is a growing trend to ask consultants to remain on site in the early hours of the evening when they are on call in medical and surgical specialties, and this should be investigated when applying for any job.

Skills and objectives

Every post will have a list of skills given within the person specification. These will be divided into 'essential' and 'desirable', so find out which of these skills you have before applying. Essential skills will include (in the UK), General Medical Council registration, completion of specialist training, and the ability to perform procedures as needed. Desirable skills may include a higher research degree, with evidence of teaching and management. When you apply for the post it is key that you are able to prove that you have as many of the desirable skills as possible.

The post will also have a series of objectives, such as to augment a rapidly growing clinical need or to start up a new clinical service. Familiarise yourself with these objectives, and with the future goals of both the Trust and the department, before applying.

Researching the Trust

Find out as much as you can about the NHS Trust before you apply. A Trust in serious financial difficulties will definitely be harder to work in than one with cash to spare. Find out about the reputation of the Trust, the hospital, the department and your future consultant colleagues. Get information from the internet, from friends and colleagues who have worked there, and from lay people (i.e. find out how the Trust is perceived by the community).

Informal discussions

It may be helpful (and is strongly recommended) that you have informal discussions about the post prior to applying. This is different from arranging a formal visit (discussed later). The best way to achieve this is to contact the clinical lead (his or her contact details will be available on the job description). During the informal discussion – which can be over the telephone or in person – it is useful to find out *why* the job is being advertised. Would you be replacing someone who is retiring, which means you would inherit the patient load? Is it a new post? If so, why has it been advertised at this particular time?

Deciding on a 'job for life'

It used to be the case that your final post was a 'job for life'. Now, in the current climate in the UK with an evolving NHS structure, it may not necessarily be for the rest of your working life. An increasing number of hospital consultants and senior GPs are moving posts after a few years.

There are a number of reasons for this and you might find that one or more of these apply to you. You might leave because you've had a better offer, in which case your first job would merely be a stepping stone to a more suitable permanent job. You might leave after disagreements within a department.

How should I prepare for the consultant interview?

After applying for a job you will have a limited time in which to prepare. You need to do a number of things before you are shortlisted. You should arrange a formal visit to the department and try to meet everyone on the interview panel. You need to research into the likely questions that come up in the interview and try to investigate and identify problems specific to the Trust. It may be helpful to have some interview practice from consultant mentors, and to arrange some mock interviews. Attending a course for this can be useful and there are an abundance of these online (discussed later).

Visiting the department

Arrange a formal visit to all of the hospital sites at which you could be working. This is important to show that you are committed to seeing exactly what the job is like. Try to find out who is on the interview panel and arrange a formal meeting (through their secretary or PA) with as many of them as possible. Often, for consultant posts, these people will be the:

- chief executive – ask about the Trust's general direction and about any sensitive issues for the Trust
- medical/clinical director – discuss any ongoing managerial problems with the department or the Trust
- clinical lead – show your departmental interest
- general manager of directorate – ask about non-clinical issues of the department and directorate
- modern matron – ask about nursing support and issues.

Researching the Trust and department

This can be done by:

- reading the Trust's annual report
- reading the latest Trust board meeting minutes (usually available on the Trust's website)

- reading the ongoing news on the website to find out what the Trust's priorities are
- reading the quality and safety accounts (from the NHS Choice website or Trust website).

Going on a course

A number of people coming up to their consultant interview go on interview preparation courses to help equip them with the necessary knowledge and techniques. These courses are usually for one or two days and are often very expensive. They are usually operated as small group sessions which allows time to practise scenarios. The key skills taught on such courses include:

- effective communication
- trying to be succinct (e.g. allowing only 2–3 minutes per answer)
- having a bullet-point approach (about three to maximum five points per question)
- announcing your message upfront and then expanding on it
- substantiating your answers
- being personal
- providing objective measures of success.

Interview practice

Mock interviews are extremely valuable, so try to have at least one before your actual interview. Invite consultants you know to a mock interview. You should try to find a dedicated time for them to do this in a quiet environment with minimal interruptions. You should take the session seriously and behave as if it were a real interview. You should also ask your mock interviewers to pretend that it is the 'real' thing too:

- Ensure you are asked difficult questions and that you are pushed to your limit.
- Keep to time.
- Try to get them to trip you up with their questioning.
- Ask for honest feedback after the process, and after the practice interview go away and reflect on these areas.

Dress code for the real day

This is a personal choice but, as with any medical interview, you should be formal, professional and exceptionally smart. Dark suits for both men and women are the safest choice and, for men, all personalised attire should be avoided (e.g. club ties). Your shoes should be polished (ideally they should be brand new) and you should not choose this moment to try out a new aftershave or perfume.

Interview questions

A number of these are very similar to the ST interview questions covered in Chapter 2, but some are more specific to consultant jobs, including:

- *Conflict/underperformance*
  - Describe a situation where you had to deal with a conflict within your team or a multidisciplinary team.
  - Describe a situation where you have dealt with a difficult colleague on a position of authority.
  - Your registrar reports to you that her junior has been late for half an hour each morning over the past three days. How do you handle the situation?
- *Team playing*
  - Outline an example of where you feel you worked particularly well as a member of a team. What did you do? Why was the team successful?
- *Management or leadership scenarios*
  - What is the difference between leadership and management in your opinion? Describe a time when you illustrated your leadership skills.
  - Describe a non-clinical situation in which you had to change the way you approached a problem in order to solve it.
  - Can you describe a time when you have successfully managed change?
- *Health economics*
  - How can you improve quality of care without increasing cost?
  - Give me an example of something you have done which improved the running of your current department.
- *What are your strengths and weaknesses?*
  - Try to pick a weakness that could also, in some scenarios, be seen as a strength, such as taking on too much or imposing high standards on your colleagues.
  - Describe a time when you were made aware of your own limitations. What did you do about it?
  - How do you handle stress?
  - How do you know that you are fit to become a consultant?

Remember that, in your interview, you need to stand out from the crowd. You may be the last candidate of the day, so try to describe experiences that are unique to you and which the panel may not be hearing for the fifth time that day. Your enthusiasm, honesty and sincerity at interview will go a long way. Importantly, while modesty is a commendable trait, no-one else can sell your attributes at this stage except you, and you should be proud to relate your achievements. This can be difficult for some people and you should therefore practise this skill.

What if I don't get the job?

It will be very downhearting if you don't get the job at the first attempt. This is made worse if you have been to several interviews without success. The key thing is to get feedback from the interview panel. A named person on the panel will be responsible for helping you with feedback and giving you advice on how to improve your skills for the next interview. As difficult as it might seem, it is vital that you listen and take heed of anything that you could improve prior to your next interview.

When you practise further mock interviews you should concentrate on these key areas of weakness. If there are things you can do to improve, then do so before your next attempt (e.g. increase your teaching commitment or improve your management skills).

The jobs market in medicine at present is tough. Remember that you have done well to make it to the interview stage, and don't lose heart. Keep on pushing and hopefully you will succeed.

What if I do get the job?

The first thing to do is pop open a bottle of your favourite drink, be it apple juice, beer or wine! After the dust has settled, it might be possible to negotiate changes to the proposed job plan before you formally accept the post. There may be small areas of concern that you want to iron out before you start, as this could be a moment when managers and consultant colleagues are more accepting than several years down the line. If that is the case, arrange an early meeting with your clinical manager, ideally before starting, so that you can finalise your job plan. You should also assess the amount of on-call work that you will be doing. Over the first few months, keep a work diary to ensure that your job plan accurately reflects the nature of your post. If it does not, then there may be scope for reducing the workload (or increasing the pay somehow), or vice versa to reflect this.

Once you have settled into your job, it is time to make the most of it. That is discussed in Chapter 14.

Sources of further information

BMJ careers: www.bma.org.uk/careers

Dr Foster: www.drfosterhealth.co.uk

NHS Choices: www.nhs.uk

NHS Jobs: www.jobs.nhs.uk

14

Now you're at the top ... what next?

Key aims of this chapter

- Helping you to choose the right senior post
- Avoiding early problems as a senior doctor
- Making the most of a consultant career.

Introduction

You have achieved that elusive ST post, and you are on your way. But where are you going? It is not unusual for a trainee doctor to slog through the professional mire, pass all the right exams, do a good fellowship, get a consultant post and then sit back and say: 'I'm here now – is this it, for the next 30 years?'

That makes your ST years very important. They are not just about impressing your immediate boss, or getting through the week. Your training programme is not meant simply to prepare you for your exit exam, but is there to furnish you with the skills to perform the role of a modern day consultant effectively.

You can be forgiven for being apprehensive about this. We have seen more changes in the role and expectations of consultants in the NHS over the past 10 to 15 years than ever before. There has never been such momentous change in the NHS, both contractually and clinically, since its inception. Many colleagues can be negative about the abilities of trainees nowadays, so much so that some of you will actually believe that you would not make a good consultant. This is, of course, nonsense. Even with more limited hours, and more restrictions on the role juniors play in the workplace, there are still 10 years of a 48-hour week to be trained. That's about 20 000 hours of training opportunity, even without reading a medical book in your spare time! If it is used effectively by your trainers, and importantly by you as the trainee, that gives you ample time to train to be a consultant.

Your first steps as a senior doctor

A change in attitude

The main challenge nowadays is to get specialist trainees into the mindset required of a consultant and for them to embrace the responsibilities borne in this role. In the past, when registrars and senior registrars were not infrequently left alone to get on with it, and 'learn by their mistakes', they acquired this mindset early on in training. Now that clinical practice at the coalface is more often delivered by consultant-grade doctors, and patients are not prepared to tolerate the 'learning by mistakes' method, coupled with many changes in the way we communicate at work, and with our colleagues and teams, this has to be taught rather than just absorbed. In our view the best way to describe this attitude is with the words:

THE BUCK STOPS HERE.

On becoming a consultant

As a trainee you work in a very structured environment, where communication with seniors and colleagues about almost every decision is built into the organisational strategy. This interaction is a vast improvement on unsupervised juniors 'having a go', especially from the point of view of the patients; but it does foster a dependence on collective or subservient decision making that can make the transition to a consultant post both challenging and stressful.

Why should that be? It is partly because, when you finally get to be 'the name over the bed', you suddenly find patients, nurses, families, other professionals and juniors all looking to *you* to provide definitive solutions to their problems. The clue is in the name – 'Consultant'! So, you have to prepare yourself in your training years to become comfortable and confident with such interactions.

Saying 'I'll discuss that with the boss' is usually acceptable when you are a trainee; but if that is your constant mantra, it will be difficult for you to adapt to the situation when you are the decision maker. That is *not* to say you should never again use the phrase 'I don't know'. Some of the most dangerous 'professionals' encountered are those who don't want to admit to a patient or colleague that they don't know or understand something, and use complicated language, 'pseudo diagnosis' or frank lies in an attempt to cover up their ignorance.

Making the most of your training years

For most trainees there will come a time when you are ready to face unfamiliar as well as common situations, and use your training, experience and professional nous to come up with a sensible and safe strategy, even if the immediate 'right answer' is not apparent, or unknown. So, during your training years:

- Make the most of all opportunities for taking on clinical and organisational responsibility.
- Try to formulate your own solution, plan or pathway to a problem before you seek the boss's opinion. If their solution is different, try to understand and question why that is. Always analyse the reasons behind a clinical action, rather than merely learning a protocol.
- Consider roles where you are given more space and responsibility before you start your consultant post; for example, clinical fellowships either as a year out of your training programme, or even after your certificate of completion of training (CCT) date.

By embracing these strategies, and acquiring the knowledge and clinical skills required to be an effective doctor, you will lay the bedrock for a successful consultant practice.

Choosing the right role

One of the wonderful things about a medical career is the plethora of opportunities. There is a niche for almost every personality type. Although you have now nailed your colours to a pathway of specialist training, keep an open mind as to whether it is right for you, and always re-evaluate your professional development plan in the context of your life plan and work–life balance as you move up the career ladder.

This applies not only to which specialty or subspecialty you choose to follow, but within that, where you choose to work, what type or size of organisation you work in, and how you develop your role as your career matures.

One of the real losses of opportunity in the recent revisions of early-years training was the potential to introduce more flexibility into career pathways.

We now have a more rigid structure of training, where it is quite difficult for young doctors to gain a purposeful experience of what actually goes on in a particular specialty or subspecialty as they are shoehorned into various 3- or 4-month F1 or F2 posts. Trainees therefore not uncommonly choose a career pathway based on a medical school memory and a short 'taster'.

That said, changing direction or having a 'portfolio career' is now not necessarily seen as 'weakness', so opportunities do exist to change path effectively. Another important consideration is that we will all tend to be working longer, so it is very important to ensure you end up in a niche that is right for you. Potentially you could be there for 30 years or more.

Here is some further food for thought:

- Think carefully about the role you will be working in as a consultant, not just picking the job that was exciting as a trainee. We all have different reasons for picking a career path – an inspiring teacher or mentor, a particular interest in a clinical aspect, a successful taster or attachment, even thoughts of financial security or intellectual plaudits! A more pragmatic reason is not always a poor motivator, but to succeed and be happy you have to have a close affinity with the choice you make.
- Look closely at the career structure and its future prospects. Many cardiothoracic surgery trainees were recently caught out by the growth of interventional cardiology and radiology; the point being that there is little point planning a career in a clinical area that is overtaken by new developments and made obsolete. Similarly, many trainees seem to be choosing general practice now, with the stated reason commonly being 'no on-calls'. However, for how long will that continue now that primary care commissioners will have to pay for emergency attendances at hospital? So, although by picking general practice you got the career you chose, you might not have got the job you wanted!
- Examine your own personality type and life goals. Are you convinced that these fit with the role you are aiming for, and will your aspirations survive the challenges and pitfalls on the way there? Have you had a chance to test these aspirations?
- Speak to as many people in – or connected to – the specialty you have chosen to discover as much about the role as you can. Understand that there are cynics, pessimists, optimists and realists out there, so always take time to evaluate the information you are given, and try to see the context of the person who has given you the information. Try to expose yourself to groups of specialists and trainees in the specialty by

attending local and national specialty group meetings to get a feel for what goes on and whether it enthuses you.

- Support your fellow trainees on the way up. Your peer group will be the people examining and evaluating your practice in the future, and will be the people you pick up the telephone to speak to when a challenge or problem presents itself. Earn and foster their respect and friendship.

Settling on that final job

The jobs market has become very competitive in recent years, following the heady days of rapid expansion in consultant numbers in the 'nineties and noughties'. Although there is a limit to how much people will compromise in choosing where they work, and with many professionals having to balance the competing interests of a partner or family careers, it is beneficial to cast the net as wide as you can in choosing the type, size and geography of the organisation you choose to settle in.

Every unit will afford different opportunities for career development; and even if you find your aspirations restricted by facilities in a certain unit, there is always the opportunity to move on in a different phase of your career. Consultant mobility, while still much less than in other professional careers, is less of a problem, unless you are seen to move regularly or frequently – which will often raise eyebrows.

The current environment makes it very difficult for a trainee to say: 'I will only be a consultant in the South West of England', or 'I will only consider working in a large city-centre teaching hospital', or 'I want to work only at Musgrove Park Hospital and settle my family in Taunton'. You need to be flexible and have a plan B. Although smaller subspecialties may demand that you work in bigger units, remember that these jobs may come up relatively infrequently. So, if Aberdeen is the closest to the role you want, then even though you trained in Bristol, you may need to apply, and discover the new wonders that a new life in the Granite City might bring!

Try to be cautious, canny and sanguine about the 'reputation' of a unit. Assess your ability to grow in an exciting and formative role in a unit that is on the up, against the established centres of excellence that may rest on their laurels and where you might find it harder to establish yourself. However, don't overestimate your ability to build a career in a unit against national trends in centralisation and commissioning imperatives – know the politics of the national and regional health economy. There are some roles that will need to be concentrated in a large teaching unit, so if you want to follow that route make sure you are knowledgeable about how teaching hospitals work!

Examine the parts of the role you aspire to, and the individual importance of each to you. Each unit or organisation, its structure and geography, will deliver a different combination of these parts, with variable emphasis in each, and it is important you match them to your aspirations. Box 14.1 will give you some pointers.

So, think long, hard and carefully about the role to which you aspire. Enjoy your aspirations and the challenges on the pathway to get there. Remain flexible and always have a plan B. Once you have confirmed your aspiration, apply, fight hard and fair, and enjoy the success of your appointment!

- Clinical exposure and demands of the job plan
- Population density, catchment area and pathology of local population
- Demographic of the unit – number of colleagues, stage of their careers and likely changes in demographic
- Opportunities to train – training rotations, fellows, educational supervision, support for regional and national training programmes such as advanced trauma life support (ATLS)
- Support structures available – radiology and pathology special interests, functional multidisciplinary teams, ITU/HDU support, wards, specialist nurses or allied health professionals
- Interaction and cooperation (or competition!) with neighbouring units – functional informal or managed clinical networks
- Career development and pastoral support – opportunities and funding available for study and professional leave, continuing medical education (CME), mentoring, appraisal
- Research opportunities – output of the hospital R&D and the unit
- Opportunities for independent practice
- Fabric of the hospital – working environment, offices, clinics, wards, theatres (even car parking and transport links)
- Postgraduate centre, conference and library facilities
- Local town, schools, housing, access to your favourite sports and activities

Box 14.1 Features of the job to consider

Now you're at the top ...

Avoiding early problems

Remember that a consultant job is a marathon, not a sprint. One of the best things about a UK consultant post is that you join a mixed team of colleagues. The best teams show a functional and dynamic blend of the wise experienced old heads and the enthusiasm and new ideas injected by younger appointments. The latter enthuse and reinvigorate the former, with the old heads acting as mentors, support and advisors to the Young Turks. This is, in our opinion at least, far better than the hierarchical structures of senior and junior consultants that exist in many other countries, and encourages a real partnership approach, rather than a parochial or dictatorial 'this is how we have always done things, so that is what you will do too'.

As a reader of this book you are likely to be at the younger end of this dynamic. It is therefore important for you to consider the best way to fit into this team structure.

Public organisations change slowly, and those working in them often change their opinions even more slowly, so a bad impression in the early years will be repented at leisure, and a careful effort to lay the proper foundations for a post will stand you in good stead for the challenges ahead. Here are some tips:

- Remember that you are a new member of the team. That team has structures, team members and ways of working that demand respect from new incumbents. Don't feel self-conscious that it takes you some time to get up to speed. Don't immediately strive to impress or overtake other members of the team to carve or enhance your reputation – that is all about satisfying your own personal significance, rather than helping develop the team, and usually ends up badly. The team appointed you because they felt you were the best person for the post; enjoy that affirmation of your abilities, and let the team help you to develop your role over time.
- Don't rely on hierarchy to cement your position on the team. The days of the traditional Professor Lancelot Spratt consultant, able to bark orders at other professionals to get what they want, are happily past. As a consultant you are by definition an articulate, intelligent and successful professional. You will have a certain amount of self-confidence that can make even very experienced colleagues from other

professions feel uncomfortable or threatened. Listen to what these colleagues have to say, go out of your way to involve them, respect their views, seek their opinion. They have lots they can teach you about the organisation and team you have joined.

- Do suggest and introduce the new ideas that will be brimming from your freshly educated mind. You may be allocated a senior mentor; if not, seek one out to help channel and control your natural enthusiasm.
- Be friendly, polite, optimistic, enthusiastic and kind. This especially applies to those who may find you intimidating – junior staff, nurses, secretaries and administrative staff for example. They are the oil that makes the engine of the unit run smoothly. They want to help you. Respect them and encourage them to want to work with you towards your goals. You cannot force them to do your bidding.
- Take part in social events, but don't go wild. Don't hang around the junior doctors' mess any more – even if you think you are cool, you will no longer be welcome.
- Make sure you pull your weight right from the start, and try to say 'yes' rather than 'no'. Be careful, however, about taking on so much that you find it difficult to cope.
- Don't be threatened or afraid of seeking advice. This has been an area of huge improvement in the past 25 years of the NHS, where the individualistic approach of 'I do, therefore I am' has been replaced by teams much happier to communicate, both within your immediate unit and on a regional and national basis. However, also have confidence in your ability to make decisions, and understand the grey areas of your field – don't feel you must have a second opinion for every difficult or controversial decision. If you have taken a proper history, conducted a thorough examination, investigated appropriately, and discussed all the management options with the patient and family, you will probably arrive at a decision that most of your peers would second and support.

Job planning

Probably the area most open to early conflicts is the 'Job Plan'. Although the NHS is much better at this now, it is still often the case that a clear job plan is not available or overt at the time of advertising and job appointment. Make sure you see a copy of your job plan before you start in post, make sure it is comprehensive, and question any holes or ambiguities. If there is an area of dispute, then clarify why it is a problem, and what the mechanism is for resolving it. Once your job plan is agreed then it is contractually binding and can be changed only by mutual agreement.

Those responsible for altering your job plan will have many competing interests to balance, and will often be under intense pressure to deliver a unit strategy. Try to be flexible, and try to see organisational development in a wider context than just your own role. That does not mean you can't or shouldn't explore why your job plan is changing and express any concerns about the adverse effects of any changes – minute and record any conversations you have about job plans and try to get all relevant information in writing. The British Medical Association (BMA) is your trade union and your industrial protection; if you are a member (and as a consultant it is advisable to join) then ask their advice on contracts, working patterns and job planning.

We will discuss developing a private practice later, but it is a common area of conflict and an area where you are relatively more exposed in the early part of your career. Don't feel you have to rush into it, and certainly don't give the impression that you are more interested in developing your independent practice than your NHS practice.

Clinical problems

Seek support for the most difficult cases rather than trying to deal with them all on your own. Even the most experienced doctors struggle with some clinical situations, and feeling out on a limb can be a very uncomfortable place when you don't have the years of experience behind you. Make sure you have a mentor, as his or her help will be invaluable in these situations.

Administration

Be thorough, prompt and meticulous with your administration. It is the basis of how you communicate with patients and other professionals, and how you record your decisions and thoughts.

Note-keeping should be legible, contemporaneous and complete. A properly filed and orderly case record, whether on paper or computer-based, is the basis for clinical communication. Make sure all relevant parties, including the patient, are copied into such communications. It is also now a GMC recommendation that all letters be copied to patients, and this should encourage you to develop a communication style that avoids medical jargon and the cardinal sin of being rude about patients in the notes. It also details a clear plan that everyone can understand.

Don't ignore piles of admin on your desk. It will annoy your secretary, GPs and other professionals who are waiting for answers and decisions, and it keeps your patients waiting longer.

Information technology (IT) can be a great help. There are, for example, picture archiving and communication systems (PACS) for radiology, computerised ordering of investigations and results, digital dictation, patient databases, and so on. Picking your way through the way the NHS does IT can be frustrating – keep calm, and get to know your local IT gurus!

Making the most of your senior career

Finding a niche

Once you are 'bedded in' – and this will vary in time for different people – you will start to feel more confident and comfortable in your role. While some people enjoy this feeling, and continue for a long time without changing further, the very personality traits that drove you to become a consultant often drives you further.

It is therefore unlikely that your role in your infancy as a consultant will satisfy you for your entire 30-year career, so use the appraisal and personal development structures available to keep reinventing your career aspirations.

The ways in which your career can develop are endless, even though many people focus on developing the clinical side of their career. There are some common areas you can look at when considering taking your career forward, both inside your unit and on a wider stage (Box 14.2).

Remember that you will sometimes have to move out of one area to allow another to develop. Also remember that the more you take on in the fields outside clinical practice, the more pressure is put on you, your family and your colleagues. Try to involve them in your planning and decisions, listen to their advice, and carry them with you because you will need their support and help. Be realistic about what each involves. If you are studying for a higher degree in biomechanics, for example, it is unlikely you will be able to obtain a masters in medical education at the same time!

Appraisal

Appraisal is now a firmly entrenched and largely very positive part of medical practice. As a trainee doctor, you will have begun to experience appraisal, if only having to learn a definition to trot out at interviews!

Most trainees are now expected to maintain a professional portfolio. While this might be viewed as simply another chore before your six-monthly

- Research – clinical and organisational
- Audit
- Evidence-based practice
- Development and evaluation of new techniques
- Developing new organisational pathways
- Teaching, training and examining
- Appraisal and mentoring
- Unit management – clinical leads and directors, leadership roles
- Committee roles – ethics, pharmaceuticals, IT, governance
- Work with professional bodies – GMC, royal colleges, subspecialty meetings both internationally, national and regionally
- Medical politics – BMA, Department of Health
- Health service organisational roles – commissioning, regional and local Trust management, liaison between primary and secondary care
- Medico-legal work – clinical negligence, CQC work
- Medical writing
- Further education – higher degrees
- Voluntary or charity work
- Overseas aid and development
- Sabbaticals and fellowships in specialist units, home or abroad

Box 14.2 Areas to consider to take your career forward

record of in-training assessment (RITA) or meeting, understanding the value of a portfolio, and getting used to keeping it up to date and relevant when you are a trainee, will stand you in very good stead for when you start your consultant post. A portfolio should include several key areas (Box 14.3).

While appraisal has often been seen in the past as a 'cosy chat' between colleagues, or even as a chance to berate a maverick or unpopular consultant, the training and support for appraisers themselves is now much better. An increase in practices such as regular '2 doctor' appraisal, involving at least one from outside the subspecialty or peer group of the appraisee, has improved the experience and made it a more useful process in guiding and supporting practice.

Revalidation

If those reading this chapter are as confused as the authors about what revalidation will finally consist of and deliver, then we are in good company!

- Job plan
- Examples and evidence of good medical practice, satisfying the domains described by the General Medical Council on clinical care, maintaining practice, relationships with patients, trainees, colleagues, probity and health: www.gmc-uk.org/guidance/good_medical_practice/contents.asp
- Summaries and evidence of all continuing medical education (CME) activity, including certificates
- Summaries and abstracts of audit and research publications or ongoing projects
- Evidence of outcome statistics, complication and/or mortality/morbidity rates associated with treatment/intervention
- A 360-degree feedback process form involving colleagues and patients
- Examples of learning from practice experience – analysis of serious untoward incidents, complications, complaints
- Personal development plan – short-, medium- and long-term
- Analysis of support and resources available and required to achieve the goals in the personal development plan

Box 14.3 Key features for your portfolio

However, the GMC does seem to have begun to better explain the system and establish how it will work.

Essentially, revalidation is a method of regulating doctors that is designed to reassure patients that we are up to date and fit to practise. Doctors revalidate by having regular appraisals. Each NHS organisation has to appoint a 'responsible officer' to ensure that the process of revalidation occurs, based on sound appraisal, in their organisation.

Based on doctors' appraisals, the responsible officer will make a recommendation to the GMC that a doctor's licence to practise should be revalidated. This will normally happen every five years.

Setting up a private practice

While this would appear one of the most attractive parts of consultancy, and for those who choose to undertake independent practice it can deliver significant rewards, it is an area fraught with difficulties and potential pitfalls for the young consultant.

It is important to consider whether one will undertake private practice at all, because there are some specialties where it is simply not feasible as the work is not out there. The local health economy is extremely variable, so if you are considering starting you need to do some research to ensure there is a market, or that one can be developed. With the increasing pressure on NHS services, and less ideological antipathy to the involvement of the private sector in healthcare in general, there is no doubt opportunities are opening up in many clinical areas.

You need to consider the demands a private practice would place on your family, NHS practice and other commitments. Interesting developments over the past decade have been limited-liability partnerships, incorporated practitioners, and group practices. These can provide opportunities to undertake independent practice while sharing some of the risk and workload. However, they rely very much on good relationships between colleagues, good communication, and very clear contracting. If you are thinking of joining such a practice, or setting one up yourself, take independent professional advice from an accountant and a lawyer with experience of corporate practice in healthcare.

The overheads of private practice are considerable. You will need a good secretary and/or practice manager, rooms (usually, but not always, in a private hospital or wing), admitting rights at one or more private facilities, and a good accountant. Remember that, as the revenue starts coming in, you will have to pay more tax as well as overheads, so it is a good idea to save or invest at least half of your income in the early years to avoid a nasty shock from the Inland Revenue!

A key overhead is *indemnity insurance*. Although some NHS patients treated in private facilities are now covered by Crown Indemnity, the vast majority of private and medico-legal practice will require separate cover. This is very important, as no matter how careful your practice, a significant complication can always arise, and subsequent litigation can be extremely costly and stressful. While many doctors stay with the larger medical defence organisations (MDOs), they do not always have the individual practitioner's reputation as their core interest, and they certainly do not offer any positive incentive to those practitioners who don't attract litigation. It can seem galling to pay very large sums of money to essentially fund those who attract the most litigation. An increasing trend in recent years is for doctors with demonstrable good outcome statistics, safe practices and lower complication and litigation rates to set up separate indemnity schemes, with potential for significant savings on premiums – so shop around!

Do not underestimate the potential for financial conflict to sour relationships. The UK has a fairly unique position where private practice is viewed by a significant proportion of doctors, and a not insignificant number of NHS workers in general, as something that is at best unseemly, and at worst immoral. If we consider the other major health economies around the world, where healthcare is largely just another personal responsibility such as the mortgage or one's pension plan, they look at the consultants of the UK almost with pity, that we remain shackled and constrained by our devotion to the NHS behemoth, while restricting our true market worth and potential. This devotion and attachment to the NHS has, however, delivered a private sector in the UK where most consultants stick to some very worthwhile tenets and principles, as outlined below.

Principle 1: A good private practice derives directly from a good NHS practice

Although the personal relationship between GPs and consultants has been consistently and purposefully eroded over the past decade – what can be described as the 'deliberate disconnection of primary and secondary care' – GPs are still largely the 'gatekeepers' of private practice. Most health insurers will not allow their policyholders direct access to consultants, and expect them to have consulted their GP first.

So, the best way to market your private practice is to ensure that you have a well run, caring and responsive public practice, with clear pathways and contact points, a good evidence base and published outcomes. This means that, although there is a real draw to the comfortable rooms of the local private hospital as soon as you start your NHS consultant post, there is much to be said for taking time to ensure you have bedded in and started to build a good reputation in the NHS first. The local demographic of practice may not give some younger consultants any choice in this if the competition is already established.

This rule applies also at the other end of practice. Unless you have an international reputation, then once you retire as a consultant from NHS practice you might see the private referrals fall off fairly sharply, as GPs tend to believe that if you feel too old to work with public patients the same probably applies to the richer ones! This means that, if you are starting a replacement post rather than a new post, your senior retiring colleague's practice is likely to decline over a year or two, which then allows a young consultant to commence some private practice after having had a chance to become established.

Principle 2: A private practice should mirror a public practice

The populations treated in private and public hospitals may be different in their expectations, social mix, health behaviour and even outcomes, but that doesn't mean they get different illnesses or require different standards of investigation or treatment. There will be some investigations or treatments that are simply not available in our increasingly rationed NHS, but it behoves a sensible and ethical practitioner to try to deliver *exactly* the same treatment standards in private practice as one does in NHS practice.

Patients also move between the two sectors, and there will often be some national or local arrangements about how this is done fairly so as not to disadvantage either those in the NHS already, or the transferring patient. One way is to produce a small document that explains these principles to the patient, which is sent with every new appointment letter, and your secretary then gets far fewer calls from patients confused about this potentially sensitive area.

Consider the situation in the most hallowed health economy of them all, the USA, where you can crudely split the population into three groups: the 25 per cent who have comprehensive insurance or are fantastically wealthy – they get over-investigated and over-treated; the 25 per cent without any insurance, relying on public sector provision – they get practically no treatment or treatment akin to that in the developing world; and finally, the under-insured middle class, terrified of chronic illness, old age and the exclusions that brings on their health policy. Largely, in the UK, this distinction does not exist, and a patient in a private hospital gets a test or operation because it is indicated, not because it earns the practitioner extra cash.

Principle 3: Don't over-sell or under-sell yourself

While most GPs are perfectly wise to consultants 'selling themselves', it is not possible to gain referrals from someone you don't know exists! So, try to get involved in groups that deliver regional education to primary care. This has the double benefit of disseminating good practice, and getting your face and name known.

Importantly, don't make claims about your practice and its benefits in relation to your colleagues'. In addition, charge fair fees that reflect your market worth. Health insurers are increasingly aggressive towards consultants to try to keep their fees down. While you have a duty to inform a patient about your fees before treatment, don't worry about robustly challenging an insurer who tries to interfere with a doctor–patient relationship because you don't adhere to their charging structure. Patients normally come out on your side!

Some final tips on private practice

- Don't charge other doctors for your time – you never know when you will be under a colleague's knife.
- Leave time for your family and other interests too. 'All work and no play makes Jack a very dull Prozac taker.'
- Don't delegate your responsibilities too much. Remember that your private patients are paying for and expect your personal attention.
- Both you and your secretary need to be easily and readily contactable at all times.

This final chapter, and the previous ones, hopefully should set you up for a successful and challenging career in medicine. Work hard, play hard, and hopefully we can meet up one day for a cocktail on the beach at the end of our lucrative, challenging and rewarding careers. Good luck !

Sources of further information

BMA employment and contracts: www.bma.org.uk/employmentandcontracts/index.jsp
GMC revalidation: www.gmc-uk.org/doctors/revalidation/9612.asp

Index